Wyatt's

Practical Psychiatric Practice

Forms and Protocols for Clinical Use

Third Edition

Wyatt's Practical Psychiatric Practice

Forms and Protocols for Clinical Use

Third Edition

Richard Jed Wyatt, M.D.

Robert H. Chew, Pharm.D.

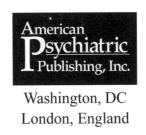

Washington, DC
London, England

Manufactured in the United States of America on acid-free paper
09 08 07 06 05   5 4 3 2 1
First Edition

Typeset in Adobe's Times New Roman and Arial

American Psychiatric Publishing, Inc.
1000 Wilson Boulevard
Arlington, VA 22209-3901
www.appi.org

Library of Congress Cataloging-in-Publication Data
Wyatt, Richard Jed, 1939–2002
    Wyatt's practical psychiatric practice : forms and protocols for clinical use / Richard Jed Wyatt, Robert H. Chew.—3rd ed.
      p. ; cm.
    Rev. ed. of: Practical psychiatric practice. 1998.
    Includes bibliographical references and index.
    ISBN 1-58562-109-9 (spiralbound : alk. paper)
    1. Psychiatry—Practice—Forms. 2. Psychiatric rating scales. 3. Patient education—Forms. I. Title: Practical psychiatric practice. II. Wyatt, Richard Jed, 1939–2002 Practical psychiatric practice. III. Chew, Robert H., 1949– IV. Title.
    [DNLM: 1. Mental Disorders—diagnosis—Forms. 2. Interview, Psychological—Forms. 3. Mental Disorders—therapy—Forms. 4. Psychopharmacology—Forms. 5. Psychotropic Drugs—Forms. WM 141 W976w 2005]
RC465.5.W94 2005
616.89—dc22

2004052945

British Library Cataloguing in Publication Data
A CIP record is available from the British Library.

Contents

Part 1: Physician Forms

INITIAL LETTER TO PATIENTS, SELF-ASSESSMENT, AND RELEASE FORMS

HISTORY AND DOCUMENTATION FORMS

RATING SCALES AND INSTRUMENTS

Part 2: Information About Psychiatric Illnesses for Patients and Families

Part 3: Information About Medications for Patients and Families

ANTIPSYCHOTICS

ANTIDEPRESSANTS

Mood Stabilizers

Antiparkinson Agents

Anti-Anxiety / Sedative-Hypnotic Agents

Agents for Treatment of ADHD

Cognitive Enhancers

Foreword

Wyatt's Practical Psychiatric Practice is the third edition of a book first published 10 years ago by my husband, Richard Wyatt. Richard was a scientist as well as a practicing psychiatrist, and he strongly believed that a scientific understanding of diagnosis and treatment should be an integral part of routine clinical care. His many years as Chief of Neuropsychiatry at the National Institute of Mental Health, as well as his long-standing and energetic involvement in mental health advocacy, made him acutely aware of the need for education not only of psychiatrists but of patients and family members as well. The extensive information for patients and family members contained in this book is a direct result of his clinical and advocacy work.

Richard was an excellent doctor. His medical degree was from Johns Hopkins, and he was powerfully influenced by the Hopkins emphasis on combining research, teaching, and clinical practice. He worked hard to put his own clinical and research expertise into a practical format that might help other doctors. I am prejudiced, of course, but I think he has done this very well. After he died in 2002, I was eager to make sure that the revision of his book was completed, and I am delighted to say that it has been, and with great skill, by Dr. Robert Chew.

Kay Redfield Jamison, Ph.D.
Professor of Psychiatry
The Johns Hopkins School of Medicine
Baltimore, Maryland

Preface to the Third Edition

For the busy clinician, *Wyatt's Practical Psychiatric Practice* manual is a convenient source for history and documentation forms, rating scales and instruments, and information handouts for patients and families about psychiatric disorders and medications. Since the release of the second edition in 1998, new antipsychotics, antidepressants, mood stabilizers, and other psychotropic agents have been introduced. Moreover, many of the older, first-generation psychotropics that were emphasized in the previous edition have been superseded by newer, second-generation agents. The revision of *Practical Psychiatric Practice* was necessary to keep up with the steady expansion of these new agents. Our endeavor for the third edition is to make it relevant and *practical* for the practitioner.

This book was conceived and written by Richard Jed Wyatt, M.D. Dr. Wyatt's passing last year left the question as to the future of his book. The editors at American Psychiatric Publishing, Inc. (APPI), believed in the unique strengths of his work. I was brought in as a consultant pharmacist to provide the redraft on the medication handouts for this book. Working with Robert E. Hales, M.D., Editor-in-Chief of APPI, we made further changes in the book to give it relevance for today's psychiatric practice. The third edition of Dr. Wyatt's *Practical Psychiatric Practice* is the result of this joint effort. True to Dr. Wyatt's intent and words, "The book is an evolving effort and will be updated periodically."

In this latest edition, the book is divided into three parts—a departure from the previous editions, which contained two parts.

Part 1 contains forms for use by the psychiatric practitioner. It includes an introductory letter that may be sent to the patient before the first visit and a self-assessment form for the patient to complete before the first visit. Other documentation forms include release of information and medical records, initial psychiatric history and assessment, a medication log, and many other forms to help organize the psychiatrist's practice. New additions to Part 1 include guidelines for clozapine prescribing and monitoring, a clozapine monitoring form, a clinical assessment and progress note (the "Patient-Physician Contact Form") for physicians to use on routine patient visits, an informed consent form, and a revised medication log.

The most significant revision in Part 1 is the deletion of several of the previous scales and instruments in the manual and the inclusion of others that we thought would have greater clinical utility—not only for their reliability and validity but also for their brevity. The 4-Item Positive Symptom Rating Scale (PSRS) and Brief Negative Symptom Assessment, the Brief Bipolar Disorder Symptom Scale, and the Quick Inventory of Depressive Symptomatology (Self-Report) (QIDS-SR) were added to the manual. They are used in the Texas public mental health system for the implementation of algorithms under the Texas Implementation of Medication Algorithms (TIMA) and are reprinted with permission from the Texas Medication Algorithm Project. Finally, the 17-item Hamilton Rating Scale for Depression (Ham-D), one of the most widely used rating scales for depression, is another addition to the book.

Researchers in the Texas Medication Algorithm Project have shown that basing therapeutic decisions on reliable, objective measures (i.e., evidence-based decisions) will ultimately enhance therapeutic effectiveness and will translate to lower medication costs and reduced hospitalization and clinic visits. Use of rating scales is pivotal in the Texas algorithm methodology in making therapeutic decisions. The researchers therefore developed abbreviated instruments that are brief and easy to administer and can be widely accepted in daily clinical practice. We believe these newly added scales and instruments will be useful for the clinician, as well.

Part 2 consists of handouts on major psychiatric illnesses that can be given to patients and families. The handouts include discussion of depressive disorders, bipolar disorder, schizophrenia, obsessive-compulsive disorder, tardive dyskinesia, and three new topics in this edition—Alzheimer's disease, anxiety disorders, and attention-deficit/hyperactivity disorder.

Part 3 consists of medication handouts for patients and families. The greatest effort was devoted to revising this section of the manual on the medication handouts. Inclusion of handouts for new drugs, as well as new handouts for drugs in other therapeutic classes (e.g., psychostimulants, cognitive disorder, benzodiazepines) that were not in previous editions, gives clinicians a total of 28 medication handouts to provide to their patients and the patients' families.

For practical purposes, when drugs could be discussed in their pharmacologic, chemical, or therapeutic class (e.g., selective serotonin reuptake inhibitors, tricyclic antidepressants, cognitive enhancers), we focused the discussion of these medications on their drug groups. The exception, however, was with the second-generation antipsychotic medications (the *atypical* antipsychotics), each of which is presented in its own handout. We believe that with the prevalent prescribing of these antipsychotics today, patients and families will want to learn more about these medications. In the previous editions, most of the medication handouts had a short and long form. This redundancy was eliminated in this edition.

Some may question if the handouts—both for psychiatric illnesses and for medications—may be too technical at the patient level. I found over the years of providing medication counseling to patients and their families that many appreciate the new knowledge they learn of their psychiatric illness and treatments. Providing this information, particularly when the information is discussed at regular intervals, is vital to "informed consent" for the prescribed treatment. As new advances in neurobiology provide greater understanding of the causes of psychiatric disorders, as well as the drugs used to treat them, I believe we have an obligation to share this knowledge and information with the patients and their families.

Moreover, the handouts may be an invaluable resource for clinicians and mental health educators as reference sheets they can provide to participants in group sessions. The points for teaching and discussion are clearly highlighted in the handouts.

ACKNOWLEDGMENTS

The third edition of *Practical Psychiatric Practice* is dedicated to the memory of Dr. Richard Jed Wyatt, the author. I wish to thank Dr. Kay Jamison for granting the copyright permission to make this edition possible. To those who provided encouragement, collaborative support, and advice, I am truly grateful. I am indebted to Robert E. Hales, M.D., Editor-in-Chief, American Psychiatric Publishing, Inc., and Professor and Chair of the Department of Psychiatry and Behavioral Sciences, University of California, Davis, School of Medicine, for taking the time from his busy schedule to provide the collaborative effort and advice on this project. I want to extend my heartfelt appreciation to Ms. Ruby Ann Lim, who spent countless hours editing the manuscript and providing insightful advice. I am also grateful to Mr. John McDuffie, Editorial Director, American Psychiatric Publishing, Inc., for putting all this together.

Robert H. Chew, Pharm.D.
Psychiatric-Pharmacist Specialist
Sacramento County Mental Health Treatment Center
Sacramento, California

About the CD-ROM

The forms and protocols are included on the enclosed CD-ROM in Adobe's Portable Document Format (PDF). The PDF files are essentially pictures of the book pages, and they will allow you to view and print the forms exactly as they appear in the book. You need Adobe's Acrobat Reader 5.0.5 or higher to view and print the PDF files; if Acrobat or Adobe Reader is not already installed on your computer, the CD-ROM will prompt you to install this free program. (Adobe Reader 6.0 is included on the CD-ROM.) Please note that you can only view and print the PDF files with the Acrobat Reader; you cannot modify them.

MINIMUM SYSTEM REQUIREMENTS—ADOBE READER 6.0

Windows

- Intel® Pentium® processor
- Microsoft® Windows 98 Second Edition, Windows Millennium Edition, Windows NT® 4.0 with Service Pack 6, Windows 2000 with Service Pack 2, Windows XP Professional or Home Edition, Windows XP Tablet PC Edition
- 32MB of RAM (64MB recommended)
- 60MB of available hard-disk space
- Internet Explorer 5.01, 5.5, 6.0, or 6.1

Macintosh

- PowerPC® G3 processor
- Mac OS X v.10.2.2-10.3
- 32MB of RAM with virtual memory on (64MB recommended)
- 70MB of available hard-disk space

GETTING STARTED

Windows

Insert the CD-ROM into your compact disc drive. The disc will AutoRun and will check to see whether Acrobat Reader 5.0.5 or higher, which is needed to open and view the files on the CD-ROM, is already present on your computer. If Acrobat Reader is *not* present, you will be prompted to install Adobe Reader 6.0. If Acrobat or Adobe Reader *is* present, you'll be presented with three choices:

- **View Main Menu**—Select this option to access the forms and protocols from the CD-ROM. Remember that you'll need to re-insert the CD-ROM each time you want to access the handouts.

- **Install Acrobat Reader 6.0**—Select this option if AutoRun alerts you that the correct version of Acrobat Reader is not installed on your computer.

- **Install files to hard drive**—Select this option if you would like to install the forms and protocols to your hard drive, instead of accessing them from the CD-ROM. You'll be asked to accept the default subdirectory for the handout files or to change to another subdirectory. Once the files are copied, double-click on **Start.pdf** from the subdirectory you specified to access the forms and protocols.

The CD-ROM uses an AutoRun feature and should start automatically when inserted into your drive. If the disc does not start automatically, or if AutoRun is disabled on your computer, from your Windows Desktop choose **Start,** then **Run,** then type the following command line: x:\autorun.exe, where *x* represents the drive letter for your CD-ROM drive.

Macintosh OS X

Insert the CD-ROM into your compact disc drive. The disc will open to display two choices (icons):

- **Read Me**—Double-click on this icon to view the installation instructions.

- **Mac OS X**—Double-click on this icon to open the folder with the Mac OS X files and indexes.

    The Mac OS X folder will list the following three choices (icons):

    - **AdbeRdr60_enu_full.dmg** —Double-click on this icon if Adobe Reader 6.0 or higher is not already installed on your computer.

    - **View Main Menu**—Double-click on this icon to access the forms and protocols from the CD-ROM. Remember that you'll need to re-insert the CD-ROM each time you want to access the handouts.

    - **Install files to hard drive**—Double-click on this icon if you would like to install the forms and protocols to your hard drive, instead of accessing them from the CD-ROM. You'll be asked to accept the default subdirectory for the handout files or to change to another subdirectory. Once the files are copied, double-click on **Start.pdf** from the subdirectory you specified to access the forms and protocols.

Macintosh OS 9

Insert the CD-ROM into your compact disc drive. The disc will open to display four choices (icons):

- **Read Me**—Double-check on this icon to view the installation instructions.

- **Install Acrobat Reader 5.1**—Double-click on this icon if Acrobat Reader 5.0.5 or higher is not already installed on your computer.

- **View Main Menu**—Double-click on this icon to access the forms and protocols from the CD-ROM. Remember that you'll need to re-insert the CD-ROM each time you want to access the handouts.

- **Install files to hard drive**—Double-click on this icon if you would like to install the forms and protocols to your hard drive, instead of accessing them from the CD-ROM. You'll be asked to accept the default subdirectory for the handout files or to change to another subdirectory. Once the files are copied, double-click on **Start.pdf** from the subdirectory you specified to access the forms and protocols.

TECHNICAL SUPPORT

Technical support is available:

    7 A.M. to 1 A.M. (EST) Monday through Friday
    8 A.M. to 8 P.M. (EST) Saturday and Sunday

Contact:

    Telephone: (888) 266-9544
    E-mail: appisupport@romnet.com

Part 1: Physician Forms

INITIAL LETTER TO PATIENTS, SELF-ASSESSMENT, AND RELEASE FORMS

HISTORY AND DOCUMENTATION FORMS

RATING SCALES AND INSTRUMENTS

Part 1: Physician Forms

INITIAL LETTER TO PATIENTS, SELF-ASSESSMENT, AND RELEASE FORMS

INSTRUCTIONS FOR USING THE INITIAL LETTER TO PATIENTS AND SELF-ASSESSMENT FORM

Most clinicians have a well-established procedure for handling their initial contact with patients. Here are some suggestions for what is often helpful to patients who are coming in for their first visit. Prior to the first appointment, consider sending an initial letter to the patient that gives the date, time, and place of the appointment. A map and directions to the office, as well as suggestions for parking and public transportation, also can be useful. Other items that can be included are a schedule of fees (including billing for missed appointments), directions for handling insurance reimbursements, and a request for the patient to fill out the *Self-Assessment Form* (Form 1–2). Calling the patient to confirm the first appointment 24 hours in advance helps decrease confusion and provides the patient with an opportunity to clear up any questions.

Occasionally, a patient will not want to receive mail that would alert others that he or she is seeing a psychiatrist. Patients can be given a chance to object to receiving such mail when they are asked for their address over the telephone. Patients are not the only ones who may feel uncomfortable with mailings. Some psychiatrists prefer to discuss fees and insurance reimbursements with patients directly or by handing out the information upon the patient's arrival at the office. Similarly, patients can be asked to fill out the *Self-Assessment Form* once they arrive at the office.

The *Initial Letter to Patients* (Form 1–1) and *Self-Assessment Form* are examples and can be modified to fit the different needs and sensibilities of each physician's or clinician's practice. One way to make the mailing slightly more personal is to write a note to each patient at the end of the *Initial Letter to Patients*.

INITIAL LETTER TO PATIENTS

Dear: _____ Date: _____

Date and Time of Appointment	
Date:	Time:
Anticipated length of initial appointment: (Follow-up visits may vary)	**Minutes:**
Initial consultation fee:	**$**

Self-Assessment Form. Before your evaluation, it is important that you complete the enclosed patient *Self-Assessment Form* in as much detail as possible. Much of the information will be readily available to you, but some of it may require an effort to obtain. The information not only will be of use during your assessment, it also will help organize your thinking about your psychiatric history.

After completing the form, make a copy for yourself and bring the original to your appointment. If there is a question on the form that you do not wish to answer or cannot answer, leave it blank.

To make it possible for me to spend more time on items directly related to medical care, I request that the bill be paid at the time of your visit. If you cannot afford the fee or are not able to make the payment at the time of the consultation, please discuss the issue with me during the appointment. I will be pleased to see you anyway.

Insurance. Because insurance plans have become more numerous and complex in the past few years, it has become impossible for me to monitor the status of patient claims. Consequently, it is now my policy to have patients fill out and monitor their own insurance forms. The amount of reimbursement from the insurance company will depend on your policy.

Every time a patient leaves the office, I give him or her a "routing slip" that includes the diagnosis and/or symptoms and the services provided. (Sometimes this routing slip has to be mailed.) You should attach the routing slip to your insurance reimbursement form and send it directly to the insurance company. If questions or problems arise during your application for reimbursement, I will try to help you with them.

I am looking forward to meeting with you.

Sincerely,

SELF-ASSESSMENT FORM

Please Print

Name	Date
Street	**Suite/Apt. #**

City	State	Zip code

Phone (home)	Phone (work)

Name of person with whom you live	Relationship

Age	Date of birth (day/month/year)

Name of person to call in an emergency	Relationship

Street	**Suite/Apt. #**

City	State	Zip code

Phone (home)	Phone (work)

Name of person filling out this form (if not patient)

Name of referring or responsible physician/clinician

Street	**Suite/Apt. #**

City	State	Zip code

Phone (home)	Phone (work)

Check those that apply.

Race					
Caucasian	❏	African American	❏	Asian American	❏
Hispanic	❏	Native American	❏	Other	❏

Religion					
Protestant	❏	Catholic	❏	Jewish	❏
Muslim	❏	Hindu	❏	Other	❏

Residence					
House	❏	Apartment	❏	Room	❏
Dormitory	❏	Hotel	❏	Hospital	❏
Other					❏

Gender		Marital Status			
Female	❏	Never married	❏	Living cooperatively	❏
Male	❏	Married	❏	Divorced	❏
Occupation		If married, how many times?		If divorced, how many times?	
		1 2 3 Other		1 2 3 Other	
		Separated	❏	Widow/widower	❏
		Marriage annulled	❏	Other	❏

Education (please specify highest level completed)		
High school and earlier (circle one)	College/university (circle one)	Graduate school (circle one)
6th or earlier 7th 8th 9th 10th 11th 12th	1 2 3 4 5 Other	BA BS MA MS MBA PHD Other

Please state the principal reason you are requesting a consultation or treatment.

_____

_____

_____

_____

_____

_____ If necessary, use another sheet of paper.

Please describe your illness from the time of your first symptom to the present. Provide as many dates, names, and addresses of psychiatrists, psychologists, and/or social workers who have treated you as you can. Also, please provide the kinds of treatment you have received, including names of medications and your response to them.

_____

_____

_____

_____

_____

_____

_____

_____

_____

_____

_____

_____

_____

_____

_____

_____

_____

_____

_____

_____

_____

_____

_____

_____

_____

_____

_____

_____

_____

_____

_____

_____

_____

_____ If necessary, use another sheet of paper.

Suicide		**Comments**
Check if you have ever thought about suicide.	❏	
If "yes," when was the last time?		
Check if you have ever attempted suicide.	❏	
If "yes," when and how?		
Check if you have thoughts about suicide now.	❏	

Injury to Others	
Check if you have ever thought about hurting someone else.	❏
If "yes," when was the last time?	
Check if you have ever hurt someone else.	❏
If "yes," when and how?	
Check if you are thinking about hurting someone now.	❏

Recent Stressful Life Events Check any of the following events that have occurred during the last 2 years.	
Married	❏
Engaged	❏
Separated	❏
Divorced	❏
Serious argument	❏
Breakup of important relationship	❏
Child left home	❏
Death of spouse, other	❏
Bad health (behavior) of family member	❏
Difficulties with family member	❏
Personal injury, illness	❏
Sexual difficulties	❏
Difficulties, changes at school, work	❏
Retired, lost job	❏
Changed residence	❏
Legal difficulties, multiple traffic tickets	❏
Owe money	❏

Drinking (Alcohol Use)

How many drinks do you consume in the average day?

At what time of day do you have your first drink?

What is the most you have had to drink in a 24-hour period during the last year?

Check if you ever felt that you were, or someone told you that you were, drinking too much? ❏

    If "yes," under what circumstances?

Drugs of Abuse
Check if you have taken any of the following drugs.

None	❏
Marijuana	❏
Amphetamines/speed	❏
Heroin/opiates	❏
PCP	❏
LSD/hallucinogens	❏
Cocaine/crack	❏
Barbiturates/sedatives/downers	❏

If you checked one or more of the drugs, under what circumstances did you take it(them)?

When did you most heavily use drugs?

When was the last time you took such drugs?

Personal History
Check any items that apply to you and explain.

Mother's pregnancy with you was abnormal	❏
Mother's delivery of you was abnormal	❏

Check if during childhood you—

were afraid to go to school	❏
had difficulty w/ reading, writing, or arithmetic/math	❏
were truant	❏
failed or repeated a grade	❏
had frequent falls	❏
were awkward at games	❏
wet bed after age 5	❏
had tics	❏
had trouble with eyes	❏
were (are) left handed	❏
mispronounced words, had a lisp, stutter/stammer	❏
had nightmares, disturbed sleep, fear of the dark	❏
ran away from home	❏
were cruel to animals	❏
often lied to families or others	❏
set fires	❏
moved often	❏
were exposed to incest	❏
were promiscuous	❏

Comments

_____

_____

_____

_____

_____

_____

_____

_____

_____

_____

_____

_____

_____

_____

_____

_____

_____

_____

_____

_____

_____

_____

_____

_____

Family History			Major Illnesses
Name	Age[a]	Occupation[b]	List all major illnesses, including psychiatric, neurological, alcoholism, drug abuse, suicide, and suicide attempts.
Mother			
Father			
Brothers			
Sisters			
Children			
Grandparents, uncles, and aunts (relationship)			

[a]Or if deceased, age at death.
[b]Or if deceased, cause of death.

13

Medical History
Weight and Height
What is your current weight in pounds?   lb.
Check if your weight has increased or decreased by more than 10 pounds during the last 5 years.   ❑
If checked, explain circumstances.
What is your height in inches?   in.
Sleep
Check if you—
have difficulty falling asleep   ❑
have difficulty waking up and falling back to sleep   ❑
are tired on waking   ❑
have bad dreams, wet bed, sleepwalk, or other sleep disturbances   ❑
Smoking
Check if you smoke.   ❑
If checked, how much and for how long?
Caffeine
Check if you drink coffee, tea, or colas.   ❑
If checked, how much?
Check if you believe you are sensitive to caffeine.   ❑
Allergies
List all allergies. Be sure to include medication allergies.

Comments

_____

_____

_____

_____

_____

_____

_____

_____

_____

_____

_____

_____

_____

_____

_____

_____

_____

_____

_____

_____

_____

_____

_____

_____

Medical Problems	
Age when first occurred	List all past and present medical problems as well as any surgery or accidents.

Females—Menstrual History	
Check if your periods are irregular.	❏
If checked, explain.	
What is the duration of your periods?	
What is the date of your last period?	
Check if there is any pain or discomfort with your periods.	❏
Check if your moods, depression, irritability, or irrationality change with your periods.	❏
If checked, how?	
Check if you are taking an oral contraceptive.	❏
If checked, which one and for how long?	
If taking an oral contraceptive, check if it affects your mood.	❏

Comments

_____

_____

_____

_____

_____

_____

_____

_____

_____

_____

_____

_____

_____

_____

_____

_____

_____

_____

_____

_____

_____

_____

15

AUTHORIZATION FOR RELEASE OF MEDICAL RECORDS

To:	
Name / Agency	
Street	
City	

State		Zip code	
Phone		**Fax**	

I, _____ , born

(date of birth) _____ , request that you send a complete copy of my

(circle one or both) psychiatric/medical records to _____ , at the

above address.

Thank you,

_____   _____
Patient's signature   Date

_____   _____
Witness's signature   Date

AUTHORIZATION FOR RELEASE OF INFORMATION

To:	
Name / Agency	
Street	
City	

State		**Zip code**	
Phone		**Fax**	

I, _____ ,

authorize _____ to give and receive

information concerning my (circle one or both) psychiatric/medical records and treatment to and from

_____ , at the above address.

Thank you,

_____   _____
Patient's signature   Date

_____   _____
Witness's signature   Date

PATIENT-PHYSICIAN AUTHORIZATIONS AND AGREEMENTS

Authorizations and agreements with _____.

Please read carefully and sign. The paragraphs below contain several agreements.

For (print patient's name) _____

Medical insurance.   I authorize the medical insurance company to pay directly for the above physician's services. However, I understand that both I and the person who signs below are responsible for all my fees, includeing any fees not paid by the insurance company.

_____   _____
Patient's or parent's signature   Date

Release of information.   I authorize _____ to release information about me to the medical insurance company and the referring physician. This authorization will end if I give written instructions to _____ to that effect, which I may do at any time.

_____   _____
Patient's or parent's signature   Date

Financial responsibility.   We, the undersigned, understand and agree that each of us is responsible for the patient's fees to _____, including any fees not paid by medical insurance; that if the account is not paid when due, reasonable collection and court costs will be paid by the undersigned; that interest at the rate of 1% per month will be charged on any balance outstanding after 90 days; that we are responsible for full therapy fees resulting from appointments not kept or canceled without a 24-hour notice; that fees for outpatient services must be paid at the time services are rendered; and that the patient is responsible for filing for insurance reimbursement.

_____   _____
Patient's or parent's signature   Date

_____   _____
Responsible party's signature   Date

INVOICE FOR SERVICES RENDERED

Patient's name: _____

Diagnosis: _____

_____

_____

Date(s) of service: _____

Nature of services: _____

_____

_____

Charge: _____

FINAL COLLECTION NOTICE

Dear [patient's name]:

I am pleased that you chose me to help you with your health needs. It is important, however, that I collect money owed me so that I can serve others.

I have contacted you several times about this past due bill. If you do not contact me within 10 days, I will be forced to turn your account over to a collection agency. To avoid having your account turned over to a collection agency, you must make payments or contact me right away. As always, I will work with you to make payment arrangements, if needed.

Sincerely,

Part 1: Physician Forms

HISTORY AND DOCUMENTATION FORMS

INITIAL PSYCHIATRIC HISTORY AND ASSESSMENT

Patient Background

Name: _____

Address: _____

Phone (home): _____   **Phone (work):** _____

Age: _____   **Date of birth:** _____

Marital status: _____

Educational background: _____

Occupation: _____

Race: _____   **Religion:** _____

Gender: _____

Referral Source and Reason for Consultation

_____

_____

Chief Complaint

_____

_____

_____

_____

Present Illness

_____

_____

_____

Suicidality

	Yes	No
Has patient ever thought about suicide?	❑	❑

If "yes," when was the last time? _____

What were the circumstances? _____

	Yes	No
History of suicide attempts?	❑	❑

If "yes," how and when? _____

	Yes	No
Current suicidal thoughts?	❑	❑

If "yes," explain: _____

	Yes	No
Current suicidal command hallucinations?	❑	❑

If "yes," explain: _____

Injury to Others

	Yes	No
Does patient express concern about hurting others?	❑	❑

If "yes," explain: _____

Alcohol and Drugs of Abuse

Number of drinks in an average day: _____

	Yes	No
Has patient ever felt, or been told, that he or she is drinking too much?	❑	❑

If "yes," explain: _____

	Yes	No
Has patient ever used drugs of abuse?	❑	❑

If "yes," explain: _____

Last time patient took drugs? _____

Check any drugs of abuse.			
marijuana	❑	PCP	❑
cocaine/crack	❑	LSD/hallucinogens	❑
amphetamines/stimulants	❑	barbiturates/sedatives	❑
heroin/opiates	❑	other street drugs	❑

Childhood Behavioral / Psychiatric Problems

_____

_____

_____

Family History

Family Member	Psychiatric Problems	Suicide/Attempts	Drug Abuse/Alcoholism
Mother			
Father			
Brothers			
Sisters			
Grandparents, uncles, aunts			
Children			

Medical History

Current weight : _____   **Height :** _____

Sleep difficulties

Check any sleep problems.			
difficulty falling asleep	❏	wets bed	❏
difficulty falling back to sleep	❏	walks in sleep	❏
tired on waking	❏	snores heavily	❏
early morning awakening	❏	stops breathing during sleep	❏
bad dreams	❏	falls asleep during strong emotions	❏
nightmares	❏	other (please specify below)	❏

Comments: _____

_____

Smoking and caffeine

	Yes	**No**
Does patient smoke?	❏	❏

How much does patient smoke? _____

How many cups of coffee, tea, and colas does patient drink each day? _____

If patient is sensitive to caffeine, describe reaction: _____

_____

Allergies (include allergies to medications)

Describe allergies, if any: _____

_____

Health problems

Describe current and past health problems, if any: _____

_____

_____

_____

_____

Sexual history

Describe sexual problems, if any: _____

_____

_____

Mental Status Examination

General appearance: _____

_____

_____

_____

Remarkable features: _____

_____

Attire: _____

_____

Facial expression: _____

_____

Psychomotor state: _____

_____

Abnormal movements and posture: _____

_____

_____

Social interaction and affect: _____

_____

_____

Eye contact: _____

Mood: _____

Feelings: _____

Cognition, perceptual abnormalities: _____

Consciousness: _____

Orientation: _____

Memory: *Recent:* _____

Past: _____

Remote: _____

Attention: _____

_____

Judgment: _____

_____

Insight: _____

_____

Fund of information: _____

_____

Intelligence: _____

_____

Check abnormalities that are present.			
ideas of reference	❑	rituals	❑
bizarre ideations	❑	phobias	❑
magical thoughts	❑	superstitions	❑
clairvoyance	❑	déjà vu	❑
recurrent illusions	❑	obsessive thoughts	❑
derealizations	❑	compulsive behaviors	❑
depersonalizations	❑	other (please specify below)	❑
fugue states	❑		❑

Explain: _____

_____

Hallucinations: _____

Delusions: _____

Diagnostic Impressions

Axis I: _____

Axis II: _____

Axis III: _____

Axis IV: _____

Axis V: _____

Recommendations / Plan

_____

_____

_____

_____

_____

Signature: _____   **Date:** _____

PATIENT-PHYSICIAN CONTACT FORM

Patient:		Date:
Chart no.	Gender:	D.O.B.

Physician:

Drug allergies:

Current medication(s):   None: ☐

_____

_____

_____

Depot medication: _____ **Date given:** _____ **Next due:** _____

Side effects to medication(s):   None: ☐

_____

_____

_____

Adherence to taking medication(s):   ☐ poor   ☐ fair   ☐ good

Mental Status Exam

Appearance: _____

Speech: _____

Affect: _____

Psychomotor activity: _____

Thought process: _____

Thought content: _____

Suicidal ideation / plans: _____

Homicidal ideation / plans: _____

Insight   ☐ poor   ☐ fair   ☐ good
Judgment   ☐ poor   ☐ fair   ☐ good

Medical conditions / findings:

Progress Notes

Diagnosis

    Axis I: _____

                   _____

    Axis II: _____

    Axis III: _____

    Axis IV: _____

    Axis V: _____

Treatment Plan

_____

_____

_____

_____

_____

_____

_____

_____

_____

_____

_____

_____

_____

_____

_____

_____

_____

_____

_____

Signature: _____ **M.D.**   **Date:** _____

INSTRUCTIONS FOR USING PSYCHOTHERAPY (TREATMENT) FOLLOW-UP NOTES

The *Psychotherapy (Treatment) Follow-up Notes* (Form 1–10) is to be used as documentation for third-party payers. Additionally, some may find it useful for organizing thoughts about a patient's treatment goals and his or her progress toward achieving them. Many clinicians will probably find that they need to modify the *Psychotherapy (Treatment) Follow-up Notes* to fit their practice, but the form should provide a model for the type of information that insurance companies and other third-party payers often request. With sufficient input from those who use this form, I hope to provide a "one-form-fits-all" *Psychotherapy (Treatment) Follow-up Notes* for the next edition.

The following components seem to be the most important for documentation:

- *Document that there is a **need** for treatment.* Need is often defined in terms of a medical necessity. There must be a loss of function or an intrusion on the function or well-being of others. Some third-party payers will accept significant personal discomfort as a need for treatment, but this rationale is less likely to meet with sympathetic eyes and ears. It is usually easier to document that there is a loss of function or intrusion on the function or well-being of others than to document personal discomfort. The need for treatment must arise out of an officially recognized diagnosis found in DSM-IV-TR (American Psychiatric Association 2000) or the International Classification of Diseases (ICD; World Health Organization 1992). As noted below, being familiar with the diagnoses and codes you use most often and using them—even if you disagree with their concept—will in the long run save time and aggravation.

- *Document that you and the patient have specific goals and objectives.* This process requires that you take issues that at times may seem vague or unstructured and transform them into well-defined problems with specific goals and objectives. (Defining such goals is often a reasonable goal in and of itself early in treatment.) These goals and objectives need to be both attainable and measurable. It may be preferable to break goals into subcategories, using time as a boundary (e.g., short-, intermediate-, and long-term goals). This subcategorization is much easier to do for those who practice various forms of behavior therapy, compared with, for example, psychodynamic therapies. Nevertheless, with some thought and planning, much psychodynamic treatment can be broken down into explainable and definable chunks that can be understood by third-party payers. It should go without saying that one should avoid using jargon or words whose meaning may not be clear to someone who reads your report but may not have your level of training.

- *Document that the treatments you plan to use and are using are consistent with the patient's needs, as well as the specific goals and objectives.* Treatments that have been shown to be efficacious in controlled studies for the disorder in question tend to be more accepted, but unfortunately for many disorders, some treatments have not been subjected to rigorous clinical trials. Many treatments that we "know" can help have not been subjected to such scrutiny. Fortunately, treatments—particularly if they are not costly— that are consistent with those widely used for the disorder are often accepted by third-party payers.

- *Physician's Current Procedural Terminology* (CPT; American Medical Association 1996). I find the CPT system almost unintelligible and not consistent with the way I want to practice medicine. I dread each new mailing from Medicare or its proxy. I could easily spend as much time deciphering these mailings as I do learning about new treatments or how to better apply the treatments already available to me. Nevertheless, CPT is a reality and something most of us will have to learn to work with. Fortunately, Chester W. Schmidt Jr. and coauthors, in their *CPT Handbook for Psychiatrists,* 3rd Edition, have made understanding CPT terminology easier, but it is still not fun.

- *Continuous documentation is necessary.* Treatment notes need to be updated regularly and need to show that you are focusing on the goals and objectives. Progress toward the goals is also usually required. Remember that maintaining the status quo may be the best that we can currently offer some patients. Unfortunately, maintaining the status quo may not be reimbursable, even though without these efforts, the patient's clinical state might decline.
- *Document that you have the competence to carry out the treatments you are using.* Usually your degree will provide the necessary information. But at times a professional license number and evidence of special training may also be required.

How long does it take to complete? I find that the *Psychotherapy (Treatment) Follow-up Notes* form takes about 5 minutes to complete after a patient leaves the office. Others will find that they can fill the form out while the patient is present and make it a part of the session. Having more "check boxes" would save time but would extend the notes to a second page.

Sensitive information. If you plan to submit the *Psychotherapy (Treatment) Follow-up Notes* form or something similar to third-party payers, be careful what you include. For example, unless a sexual issue is the primary reason for the treatment, it is often best not to write about it on notes that might be read by third parties. Also, under certain circumstances your notes may be subpoenaed, or worse, they may be seized by a law enforcement agency investigating you; the latter recently happened to a colleague who was thought to be prescribing drugs recklessly (he was not). Be careful!

Storage and disposal. Store your records where unauthorized individuals cannot see them (a locked file cabinet will keep out all but the most determined snooper). When you no longer need your records, make sure you destroy them (for example, run them through a paper shredder before discarding them); do not place your records in the garbage, where someone can find them. If you are not able to destroy your records yourself, make sure that someone you trust does so. If you become incapacitated or die, you may want to leave clear instructions asking a spouse, significant other, or trusted colleague to destroy your records for you.

DEFINITIONS

[Medical] evaluation and management (EM) services involve a variety of responsibilities unique to the medical management of psychiatric patients, including medical diagnostic evaluation; drug management, when indicated; psychiatric orders; interpretation of laboratory or other medical diagnostic studies and observations; review of activity therapy reports; supervision of nursing and ancillary personnel; programming of all hospital resources for diagnosis and treatment; and activity as a leader or director of a treatment team as related to that patient.

Interactive psychotherapy is typically furnished to children. It involves the use of physical aids and non-verbal communication to overcome barriers to therapeutic interaction between the psychiatrist and the patient who has lost, or has not yet developed, either the expressive language skills to explain his or her symptoms and response to treatment or the receptive communication skills to understand the psychiatrist if he or she were to use ordinary adult language for communication.

Insight-oriented, behavior-modifying, and **supportive psychotherapy** refer to the development of insight or affective understanding, the use of behavior modification techniques, the use of supportive interactions, the use of cognitive discussion of reality, or any combination of the above to provide therapeutic change.

A **consultation** indicates that no treatment has taken place but that there has been communication with a referring health care provider.

Modifiers to CPT codes. When the activity (oftentime) associated with the procedural code is not adequate to describe what was actually done, it may be appropriate to use modifier codes. These two-digit codes follow the traditional five-digit code separated by a hyphen.

- **-21   Prolonged Evaluation and Management Services.** When the service unit is greater than that covered by the highest level of service covered by the traditional code, use the -21 suffix.

- **-25   Significant, Separately Identifiable Evaluation and Management.** When a service is provided by the same psychiatrist on the same day as another procedure or other service and it was necessary to perform that service on the same day as a previous service, use the -25 suffix.

- **-32   Mandated Services.** When services were mandated by a third party, such as the payer, use the -32 suffix.

- **-52   Reduced Services.** When the service unit is reduced in time from the lowest level covered by the traditional codes, use the -52 suffix.

G codes. The **"G"** codes are to be substituted for previous psychotherapy service codes 90842, 90843, 90844, and 90855 when Medicare reimbursement is sought after January 1, 1997 (U.S. Government Printing Office 1996). Most third-party payers will accept the traditional codes. The new "G" codes eliminate "medical" from "medical psychotherapy" and do not include the CPT descriptor "by a physician" so that the psychotherapy "only" code can be used by psychiatrists, psychologists, and social workers.

REFERENCES

American Medical Association: Physician's Current Procedural Terminology: CPT 97. Chicago, IL, American Medical Association, 1996

American Psychiatric Association: Diagnostic and Statistical Manual of Mental Disorders, 4th Edition, Text Revision. Washington, DC, American Psychiatric Association, 2000

Schmidt CW Jr, Yowell RK, Jaffe E: CPT Handbook for Psychiatrists, 3rd Edition. Washington, DC, American Psychiatric Publishing, 2004

U.S. Government Printing Office: Federal Register, Washington, DC, November 22, 1996

World Health Organization: ICD-10 Classification of Mental and Behavioural Disorders: Clinical Descriptions and Diagnostic Guidelines. Geneva, World Health Organization, 1992

PSYCHOTHERAPY (TREATMENT) FOLLOW-UP NOTES

Patient's name	Patient no. (if any)

Activity since last visit Check as appropriate.

☐ **99371, 99372, 99373 (Telephone calls):**

☐ **Missed appointment:**

Other:

☐ **90825 (Evaluation of tests/records):**

Current therapy

Procedure codes—check one.	Date(s): Time began: A.M./P.M. Time ended:
Individual psychotherapy modifiers,	Location of session(s): ☐ Office ☐ CMCH ☐ Partial hospitalization
if used: –22 for less than amount of time;	☐ Nursing home ☐ Hospital ☐ Other
–52 for longer than amount of time	Current state (or problems) of patient:
☐ G0071	Symptoms requiring current level of care:
☐ G0072	
☐ G0073	
☐ G0074	Environmental stressors:
☐ 90862 (Medication management)	
☐ 90847 (Family therapy with pt.)	Goals of current therapy:
☐ 90845 (Medical psychoanalysis)	
☐ 90899 Not specifically defined (explain):	Response to therapy in terms of goals:
☐ Other (explain):	New issues:

Therapeutic interventions used during session: ☐ Face-to-face psychotherapy   ☐ Behavioral therapy   ☐ Other

Medical issues and test values: ☐ None

Pharmacotherapy changes: ☐ None

Issues for next session:

Level of collaboration: ☐ Least–1   ☐ 2   ☐ 3   ☐ 4   ☐ 5   ☐ 6–Most

Date of next session:

Signature / Title: Date:

INFORMED CONSENT FOR TREATMENT WITH PSYCHOTROPIC MEDICATIONS

Patient: _____   **Date:** _____

(Print)

My physician has explained to me the nature of my mental disorder, and my physician and I have decided the best course of treatment is with one or more of the following medications:

Drug class[a]	Medication	Dosage range	Route

Note. AD = antidepressant; AP = antipsychotic; AX = anti-anxiety; CE = cognitive enhancer; MS = mood stabilizer; SH = sedative-hypnotic; PS = psychostimulant; NPS = nonpsychostimulant for ADHD.

My physician has explained the reasons for taking the above medication(s), including the risks and benefits of the treatment, the likelihood of improving without medications, and other possible alternative treatments.

The most common side effects associated with the medication(s) have been explained, and I understand that other possible side effects from my medication(s) may occur. If any untoward side effect should occur, I have been instructed to promptly notify my physician or a clinic staff member. Moreover, my physician has provided me with a *Medication Information Handout(s)* for the medication(s) that I am taking.

I understand that by giving consent I am voluntarily giving permission for use of medication for treatment of my mental disorder. I also understand that there may be risks associated with my treatment, as well as benefits for treating my condition. My consent may be withdrawn at any time if I notify my physician. I also understand that discontinuation of the prescribed medication(s) without consulting my physician may result in worsening of my condition.

Signatures of the:

Patient: _____ **Date:** _____

Conservator: _____ **Date:** _____

**Parent or
Guardian:** _____ **Date:** _____

Witness: _____ **Date:** _____

Physician: _____ **Date:** _____

- -

Withdrawal of Consent:

I (or on behalf of my child / conservatee) withdraw my consent to take the above medication(s) as prescribed.

Signature: _____ **Date:** _____

Physician: _____ **Date:** _____

Reason for withdrawal of consent:

MEDICATION LOG

Start date	Medication/Strength	Frequency	D/C date	Reason medication changed or discontinued	Comments (side effects, lab results, etc.)

CLOZAPINE PRESCRIBING AND MONITORING GUIDELINES

Currently, there are three pharmaceutical companies[1] that market clozapine: Novartis Pharmaceuticals, the manufacturer of Clozaril, and Mylan Laboratories and Ivax Pharmaceuticals, which market generic clozapine. Each company employs their own registry system for monitoring, tracking, and reporting patients' white blood cell (WBC) count and the absolute neutrophil count (ANC). All registries must conduct a rechallenge status check from the National Non-Rechallenge Masterfile, which is maintained by Novartis Pharmaceuticals, on all patients who are beginning clozapine for the first time or restarting clozapine, or if a patient's clozapine history is unknown at the time of registration. The National Non-Rechallenge Masterfile is a national database that identifies patients whose reported WBC count and ANC are below critical levels, who require termination of clozapine therapy, and who should not be reexposed to clozapine. For example, if a patient's WBC count falls below 2000 per mm^3 or ANC falls below 1000 per mm^3 while taking clozapine, the values are reported to the patient's registry by the pharmacy or clinician. The registries at Ivax and Mylan must forward the patient's data to Novartis Pharmaceuticals' Clozaril National Registry for posting to the National Non-Rechallenge Masterfile. In the event the patient is re-registered for clozapine therapy, the registry representative will notify the pharmacist or physician that the patient should not be reexposed to clozapine. Thus, through the Non-Rechallenge Masterfile, a patient with a history of leukopenia or agranulocytosis can be identified, even if the patient had previously received clozapine from another prescriber and pharmacy or registered under another company.

To minimize the risk of potentially fatal agranulocytosis, clozapine therapy requires a strict monitoring system that ensures a weekly or biweekly WBC count report prior to dispensing of the next supply of medication. Each pharmaceutical company employs their own registry system, but the requirements are essentially the same. The clozapine treatment systems requirements are outlined below.

CLOZAPINE TREATMENT SYSTEMS REQUIREMENTS

A. Systems Registration

1. Each registry requires registration of the patient, dispensing pharmacy, and treating physician. The pharmacy generally registers the patient, fills out the required forms for the physician to sign, and submits the completed forms to the registry.

    *   Online information and registration are available through Novartis Pharmaceuticals' Clozaril Administration Registry Enrollment (CARE), Ivax Pharmaceuticals' Clozapine Patient Registry, and Mylan Laboratories' Clozapine Prescription Access System (CPAS).

---

[1] At the time of this writing, there are three pharmaceutical companies that market clozapine; however, another generic manufacturer may soon market clozapine as well.

B. Treatment Requirements

1. A baseline WBC count dated within 7 days prior to the dispensing date of clozapine is required, and the WBC count must be greater than 3500 per mm^3. For patients who are reinitiating clozapine and were on biweekly monitoring, a WBC count within 14 days of the dispensing date is required.

2. Once a patient is registered and his or her eligibility is confirmed, a 1- or 2-week supply of clozapine may be dispensed per physician prescription.

3. Prior to dispensing the next supply of clozapine, the pharmacist must obtain and forward the current report of the weekly or biweekly WBC count and the current total daily dosage to the patient's registry. The treating physician is responsible for ordering weekly or biweekly WBC counts, ensuring that the dispensing pharmacy receives the report. If the pharmacy did not receive the WBC count before the next dispensing date, the pharmacist must inform and consult with the patient's physician. Generally, the pharmacist dispenses the clozapine, and the physician orders an immediate WBC count.

4. Patients who are on weekly monitoring for up to 6 months of continuous therapy may have their monitoring reduced to every other week, provided that their weekly WBC counts are within normal limits (>3500/mm^3). The treating physician, of course, determines the monitoring frequency but must meet the minimum requirements of the treatment system.

C. Interruption or Discontinuation of Clozapine Treatment When:

Event	Required action	Results	Further action
WBC count is 3000–3500,[a] or dropped significantly,[b] or immature cell forms are present	Repeat WBC count and differential count; advise patient to immediately report appearance of fever, sore throat, or other signs of infection.	If repeat WBC count is 3000–3500 and absolute neutrophil count[c] (ANC) > 1500 and no immature cell forms, continue clozapine therapy.	Twice-weekly WBC count and differential until WBC count > 3500 and cell differential normal.
WBC count 2000–3000 or ANC 1000–1500	Interrupt clozapine therapy and notify registry. WBC counts with differential daily until WBC count ≥ 3000 and ANC ≥ 1500.	WBC count ≥ 3000 and ANC ≥ 1500, and no symptoms of infection are present.	May restart clozapine with twice-weekly WBC count until WBC count ≥ 3500, then WBC count weekly for 6 months.
WBC count < 2000 or ANC < 1000 ANC < 500 (agranulocytosis) with signs of infection (fever, malaise, weakness, lethargy); this constitutes a medical emergency.	Immediately and permanently discontinue clozapine. Monitor patient closely for fever and other signs of infection. Order daily tests until WBC count and differential return to normal (WBC ≥ 3500 and ANC ≥ 1500).	If WBC count > 3500, repeat posttreatment WBC count and differential weekly for 4 weeks.	Consult hematologist for treatment options. Pharmacist notifies registry of discontinuation and provides serial WBC count results.

[a]WBC count and ANC per mm^3.
[b]"Dropped significantly" is defined as a single drop of 3000 mm^3 or more, or a cumulative drop of 3000 mm^3 or more within 3 weeks.
[c]ANC/mm^3 = WBC (mm^3) × neutrophil (%). Example: If WBC = 7500/mm^3 and neutrophils = 35%, ANC = 7500 × 0.35 = 2625 mm^3.

D. Clozapine Registries

Clozaril Administration Registry Enrollment (CARE)
Novartis Pharmaceutical Corporation
One Health Plaza
East Hanover, NJ 07936
Phone: 1-800-448-5938
Fax: 1-800-368-5564
Web site: www.clozarilregistry.com/care
Online registration is available.

Clozapine Patient Registry
Ivax Pharmaceuticals, Inc.
50 NW 176th Street
Butler Building, Second Floor
Miami, FL 33169
Phone: 1-800-507-8334
Fax: 1-800-507-8339
Web site: www.clozapineregistry.com
Online registration is available.

Clozapine Prescription Access System (CPAS)
Mylan Laboratories, Inc.
Phone: 1-800-843-9915
Fax: 1-800-843-9916
Web site: www.mylan-clozapine.com
Online registration is available.

Clozapine Monitoring Form

Patient Information

Patient name: _____

Social Security #: _____

D.O.B.: _____

Allergies: _____

Diagnosis: _____

Registration Information

Physician: _____

Physician's DEA #: _____

Manufacturer: _____

Registry fax: _____

Registry phone: _____

Date	/ /	/ /	/ /	/ /	/ /	/ /	/ /	/ /	/ /	/ /
WBC / mm^3										
Neutrophils (%)										
ANC^1 / mm^3										
Platelets / mm^3										
Weight										
Clozapine dosage (mg/day)										

^{1}ANC/mm^3 = WBC (per mm^3) × Neutrophils (%).

Concurrent medications: _____

Progress notes: _____

_____

_____

42

Part 1: Physician Forms

RATING SCALES AND INSTRUMENTS

INSTRUCTIONS FOR USING THE
4-ITEM POSITIVE SYMPTOM RATING SCALE (PSRS) AND
BRIEF NEGATIVE SYMPTOM ASSESSMENT (BNSA)

INTRODUCTION

The 4-Item Positive Symptom Rating Scale (PSRS) and Brief Negative Symptom Assessment (BNSA) are instruments used by the Texas Medication Algorithm Project (TMAP) in the Texas public mental health system for assessing the symptoms of schizophrenia. The PSRS was adapted from the expanded version of the Brief Psychiatric Rating Scale (Ventura et al. 1993), and the BNSA was adapted from the Negative Symptom Assessment (Alphs et al. 1989) and the Assessment of Negative Symptoms (Andreasen 1984).

4-ITEM POSITIVE SYMPTOM RATING SCALE (PSRS)[1]

Scale Items and Anchor Points

Item 1. Suspiciousness: Expressed or apparent belief that other persons have acted maliciously or with discriminatory intent. Include persecution by supernatural or other nonhuman agencies (e.g., the devil). *Note:* Ratings of "3" or above should also be rated under Unusual Thought Content.

Do you ever feel uncomfortable in public? Does it seem as though others are watching you? Are you concerned about anyone's intentions toward you?

Is anyone going out of their way to give you a hard time or trying to hurt you? Do you feel in any danger?

[If the patient reports any persecutory ideas/delusions, ask the following:]

How often have you been concerned that [use the patient's description]*? Have you told anyone about these experiences?*

NA	**Not Assessed**
1	**Not Present**
2	**Very Mild:** Seems on guard. Reluctant to respond to some "personal" questions. Reports being overly self-conscious in public.
3	**Mild:** Describes incidents in which others have harmed or wanted to harm him/her that sound plausible. Patient feels as if others are watching, laughing, or criticizing him/her in public, but this occurs only occasionally or rarely. Little or no preoccupation.
4	**Moderate:** Says others are talking about him/her maliciously, have negative intentions, or may harm him/her. Beyond the likelihood of plausibility, but not delusional, incidents of suspended persecution occur occasionally (less than once per week) with some preoccupation.

---

[1]Reprinted with permission from Chiles JA, Miller AL, Hall CS, et al.: *Texas Implementation of Medication Algorithms (TIMA): Schizophrenia Module. Administration Manual: 4-Item Positive Symptom Rating Scale and Brief Negative Symptom Assessment*, Version 5.0. Austin, Texas Department of Mental Health and Mental Retardation, 2001.

5   **Moderately Severe:** Same as 4, but incidents occur frequently, such as more than once per week. Patient is moderately preoccupied with ideas of persecution or patient reports persecutory delusions expressed with much doubt (e.g., partial delusions).

6   **Severe:** Delusional—speaks of Mafia plots, the FBI, or others poisoning his/her food, persecution by supernatural forces.

7   **Extremely Severe**: Same as 6, but the beliefs are bizarre or more preoccupying. Patient tends to disclose or act on persecutory delusions.

Item 2. Unusual Thought Content: Unusual, odd, strange, or bizarre thought content. Rate the degree of unusualness, not the degree of disorganization of speech. Delusions are patently absurd, clearly false or bizarre ideas that are expressed with full conviction. Consider the patient to have full conviction if he/she has acted as though the delusional belief were true. Ideas of reference/persecution can be differentiated from delusions in that ideas are expressed with much doubt and contain more elements of reality. Include thought insertion, withdrawal, and broadcast. Include grandiose, somatic, and persecutory delusions even if rated elsewhere. *Note:* If Somatic Concern, Guilt, Suspiciousness, or Grandiosity are rated "6" or "7" due to delusions, then Unusual Thought Content must be rated a "4" or above.

[Ask the following:]

Have you been receiving any special messages from people or from the way things are arranged around you? Have you seen any references to yourself on TV or in the newspaper?

Can anyone read your mind?

Do you have a special relationship with God?

Is anything like electricity, X-rays, or radio waves affecting you?

Are thoughts put into your head that are not your own?

Have you felt that you were under the control of another person or force?

[If the patient reports any odd ideas/delusions, ask the following:]

How often do you think about [use patient's description]?

Have you told anyone about these experiences? How do you explain the things that have been happening [specify]?

NA   **Not Assessed**

1   **Not Present**

2   **Very Mild:** Ideas of reference (people may stare or may laugh at him), ideas of persecution (people may mistreat him). Unusual beliefs in psychic powers, spirits, UFOs, or unrealistic beliefs in one's own abilities. Not strongly held. Some doubt.

3   **Mild:** Same as 2, but degree of reality distortion is more severe as indicated by highly unusual ideas or greater conviction. Content may be typical of delusions (even bizarre) but without full conviction. The delusion does not seem to have fully formed but is considered as one possible explanation for an unusual experience.

4   **Moderate:** Delusion present, but no preoccupation or functional impairment. May be an encapsulated delusion or a firmly endorsed absurd belief about past delusional circumstances.

5   **Moderately Severe:** Full delusion(s) present with some preoccupation OR some areas of functioning disrupted by delusional thinking.

6   **Severe:** Full delusion(s) present with much preoccupation OR many areas of functioning disrupted by delusional thinking.

7   **Extremely Severe:** Full delusion present with almost total preoccupation OR most areas of functioning disrupted by delusional thinking.

Item 3. Hallucinations: Reports of perceptual experiences in the absence of relevant external stimuli. When rating degree to which functioning is disrupted by hallucinations, include preoccupation with the content and experiences of the hallucinations, as well as functioning disrupted by acting out on the hallucinatory content (e.g., engaging in deviant behavior due to command hallucinations). Include "thoughts aloud" (*gedankenlautwerden*) or pseudohallucinations (e.g., hears a voice inside head) if a voice quality is present.

Do you ever seem to hear your name being called?

Have you heard any sounds or people talking to you or about you when there has been nobody around? [If hears voice:] *What does the voice/voices say? Did it have a voice quality?*

Do you ever have visions or see things that others do not see? What about smell—odors that others do not smell?

[If the patient reports hallucinations, ask the following:]

Have these experiences interfered with your ability to perform your usual activities/work?

How do you explain them? How often do they occur?

NA   **Not Assessed**

1   **Not Present**

2   **Very Mild:** While resting or going to sleep, sees visions, smells odors, or hears voices, sounds, or whispers in the absence of external stimulation, but no impairment in functioning.

3   **Mild:** While in a clear state of consciousness, hears a voice calling the subject's name, experiences nonverbal auditory hallucinations (e.g., sounds or whispers) or formless visual hallucinations, or has sensory experiences in the presence of modality—relevant stimulus (e.g., visual illusions) infrequently (e.g., 1–2 times per week) and with no functional impairment.

4   **Moderate:** Occasional verbal, visual, gustatory, olfactory, or tactile hallucinations with no functional impairment OR nonverbal auditory hallucinations/visual illusions more than infrequently or with impairment.

5   **Moderately Severe:** Experiences daily hallucinations OR some areas of functioning disrupted by hallucinations.

6   **Severe:** Experiences verbal or visual hallucinations several times a day OR many areas of functioning disrupted by these hallucinations.

7   **Extremely Severe:** Persistent verbal or visual hallucinations throughout the day OR most areas of functioning disrupted by these hallucinations.

Item 4. Conceptual Disorganization: Degree to which speech is confused, disconnected, vague, or disrganized. Rate tangentiality, circumstantiality, sudden topic shifts, incoherence, derailment, blocking, neologisms, and other speech disorders. Do not rate content of speech.

NA	**Not Assessed**
1	**Not Present**
2	**Very Mild:** Peculiar use of words or rambling, but speech is comprehensible.
3	**Mild**: Speech a bit hard to understand or make sense of due to tangentially, circumstantiality, or sudden topic shifts.
4	**Moderate**: Speech difficult to understand due to tangentiality, circumstantiality, idiosyncratic speech, or topic shifts on many occasions OR 1–2 instances of incoherent phrases.
5	**Moderately Severe**: Speech difficult to understand due to circumstantiality, tangentiality, neologisms, blocking, or topic shifts most of the time OR 3–5 instances of incoherent phrases.
6	**Severe**: Speech is incomprehensible due to severe impairments most of the time. Many PSRS items cannot be rated by self-report alone.
7	**Extremely Severe**: Speech is incomprehensible throughout interview.

Sources of information (check all applicable):
_____ **Patient**
_____ **Parent / Relatives**
_____ **Mental health professionals**
_____ **Chart**

Explain here if validity of assessments is questionable:
_____ **Symptoms possibly drug-induced**
_____ **Underreported due to lack of rapport**
_____ **Underreported due to negative symptoms**
_____ **Patient is uncooperative**
_____ **Difficult to assess due to formal thought disorder**
_____ **Other:** _____

Confidence in assessment:
_____ **1 = Not at all to 5 = Very confident**

BRIEF NEGATIVE SYMPTOM ASSESSMENT (BNSA)[2]

Item 1. Prolonged Time to Respond (a measure of alogia): Observed throughout communications with the patient. After being asked a question, he or she pauses for inappropriately long periods before initiating a response. Delay is considered a pause if it feels as though you are waiting for a response or if you consider repeating the question because it appears that the patient has not heard you. He or she may seem "distant," and the examiner may wonder if the patient has even heard the question. Prompting usually indicates that the patient is aware of the question but has been having difficulty in developing his or her thoughts in order to make an appropriate reply. Rate severity on the frequency of these pauses.

1. **Normal:** No abnormal pauses before speaking.

2. **Minimal:** Minimal evidence of inappropriate pauses (brief but not abnormally lengthy pauses occur). May be extreme of normal.

3. **Mild:** Occasional noticeable pauses before answering questions. Because of the length of the pause, you feel the need to repeat yourself once or twice during the interview.

4. **Moderate:** Distinct pauses occur frequently (20%–40% of responses).

5. **Marked:** Distinct pauses occur most of the time (40%–80% of responses).

6. **Severe:** Distinct pauses occur with almost every response (80%–100% of responses).

Item 2. Emotion: Unchanging Facial Expression; Blank, Expressionless Face (a measure of flat affect): The patient's face appears wooden, mechanical, frozen. Facial musculature is generally expressionless and unchanging. The patient does not change expression, or the change is less than normally expected, as the emotional content of discourse changes. Because of this, emotions may be difficult to infer. Disregard changes in facial expression due to abnormal involuntary movements, such as tics and tardive dyskinesia. The two dimensions of importance when making this rating are degree of emotional expression and spontaneity.

1. **Normal:** Spontaneous displays of emotions occur when expected. Normal degree of expressiveness of emotion is present.

2. **Minimal:** Spontaneous expressions of emotion occur when expected. However, there is a reduction in the degree of emotions expressed (e.g., patient smiles only slightly when talking about something that made him very happy). May be extreme of normal.

3. **Mild:** Spontaneous expressions of emotion occur infrequently. When emotions are expressed, there is a reduction in the degree or intensity displayed.

4. **Moderate:** Obvious reduction in spontaneous expressions. Spontaneous expressions of emotions may occur very rarely during interaction and only when discussing topics of special interest or humor to the subject.

5. **Marked:** Facial expression is markedly decreased. There are no spontaneous expressions of emotion unless the patient is prompted or coaxed by the interviewer.

6. **Severe:** There are no expressions of emotions even when attempts are made to elicit an emotional response. The subject's face remains blank throughout the interview.

---

[2]Items adapted from Alphs et al. 1989; Andreasen 1984.

Item 3. Reduced Social Drive (a measure of asociality): This item assesses how much the subject desires to initiate social interactions. Desire may be measured in part by the number of actual or attempted social contacts with others. If the patient has frequent contact with someone (e.g., family member) who initiates the contact, does the patient appear to desire the contact (i.e., would he or she initiate contact if necessary?)? In making this rating, probe the desire to initiate social interactions, the number of social interactions, and the ability to enjoy them.

Assessed by asking the patient questions like:

How have you spent your time in the past week?

Do you live alone or with someone else?

Do you like to be around people?

Do you spend much time with others?

Do you have difficulty feeling close to others?

Who are your friends?

How often do you see them?

Did you see them this past week?

Have you called them on the phone?

When you get together, who decides what to do and where to go?

When you spend time with others, do you ask them to do something with you or do you wait until they ask you to do something?

Is anyone concerned about your happiness or well-being?

1   **Normal:** Normal desire to initiate any number of contacts. Social contacts are enjoyable.

2   **Minimal:** Minimal reduction in either the desire to initiate social contacts or the number of social relationships. May initially seem guarded, but has the ability to establish relationships over time. Social relationships are enjoyable.

3   **Mild:** Reduction in desire to initiate social contacts. The patient has few social relationships, and these social contacts are enjoyable.

4   **Moderate:** Obvious reduction in the desire to initiate social contacts. The patient has few relationships toward which he or she feels indifference. However, a number of social contacts are initiated each week.

5   **Marked:** Marked reduction in desire to initiate social contacts. The patient has few relationships toward which he or she feels indifference. The patient dose not initiate social contacts but may maintain a few contacts (such as with family).

6   **Severe:** Patient does not desire social contact. Actively avoids social interactions.

Item 4. Grooming and Hygiene (a measure of amotivation): Observed during the interaction with the patient. The patient displays less attention to grooming and hygiene than normal. The patient presents with poorly groomed hair, disheveled clothing, etc. Do not rate grooming as poor if it is simply done in what one might consider poor taste (e.g., wild hairdo or excessive makeup). In addition to observation, one must ask the patient about regularity of bathing, brushing teeth, changing clothes, etc. This is particularly important with out-patients, as patients may present their best grooming and hygiene at their clinic visit. Two dimensions to keep in mind when making this rating are current appearances and regularity of grooming behaviors.

Assess the patient by asking questions like:

How many times in the past week have you taken a shower or bath?

How often do you change your clothes?

How often do you shower or brush your teeth?

1   **Normal:** Patient is clean (e.g., showers every day) and dressed neatly.

2   **Minimal:** Minimal reduction in grooming and hygiene may be at the extreme end of the normal range.

3   **Mild:** Apparently clean but untidy appearance. Clothing may be mismatched. Patient may shower less often than every other day, or may brush teeth less than every day.

4   **Moderate:** There is an obvious reduction in grooming and hygiene. Clothes may appear unkempt and rumpled, or the patient may look as if he or she just got out of bed. The patient may go without shower or bathing for 2 days at a time. The patient may go for 2 days without brushing their teeth.

5   **Marked:** There is a marked reduction in grooming and hygiene. Clothing may appear dirty, stained, or very unkempt. The subject may have greasy hair or a body odor. The patient may go 3 days at a time without showering or 3–4 days without brushing teeth.

6   **Severe:** Clothes are badly soiled. Patient has a foul odor. Patient may go more than 4 days in a row without showering or more than 4 days in a row without brushing his or her teeth. Poor hygiene may present a health risk.

REFERENCES

Alphs LD, Summerfelt A, Lann H, et al: The Negative Symptom Assessment: a new instrument to assess negative symptoms of schizophrenia. Psychopharmacol Bull 25(2):159–163, 1989

Andreasen N: Modified scale for the assessment of negative symptoms. NIMH Treatment Strategies in Schizophrenia Study (ADM 9-85). Rockville, MD, U.S. Dept of Health and Human Services, Public Health Service, 1984, pp 9–102

Chiles JA, Miller AL, Hall CS, et al: Texas Implementation of Medication Algorithms (TIMA): Schizophrenia Module. Administration Manual: 4-Item Positive Symptom Rating Scale and Brief Negative Symptom Assessment, Version 5.0. Austin, Texas Department of Mental Health and Mental Retardation, 2001

The 4-Item PSRS was adapted from the Expanded Version of the BPRS developed by Ventura et al. (1993).

Ventura J, Lukoff D, Nuechterlein KH, et al: Manual for the Expanded Brief Psychiatric Rating Scale. Int J Methods Psychiatry Res 3:227–244, 1993

The Brief Negative Symptom Assessment was adapted from the Negative Symptom Assessment and the Scale for the Assessment of Negative Symptoms developed, respectively, by Alphs et al. (1989) and Andreasen (1984).

4-ITEM POSITIVE SYMPTOM RATING SCALE (PSRS) AND BRIEF NEGATIVE SYMPTOM ASSESSMENT (BNSA)[1]

Score Sheet

Patient:_____

Date:_____

4-Item PSRS Rating Scale

NA	1	2	3	4	5	6	7
Not assessed	Not present	Very mild	Mild	Moderate	Moderately severe	Severe	Extremely severe

Rate items on the basis of patient's self-reporting during interview. Item 2 is also rated on observed behavior during the interview. Item 4 is rated on the basis of observed behavior and speech.

	NA	1	2	3	4	5	6	7
1. Suspiciousness	NA	1	2	3	4	5	6	7
2. Unusual thought content	NA	1	2	3	4	5	6	7
3. Hallucinations	NA	1	2	3	4	5	6	7
4. Conceptual disorganization	NA	1	2	3	4	5	6	7

Score:_____

Brief Negative Symptom Rating Scale

	1	2	3	4	5	6	7
1. Prolonged time to respond	1	2	3	4	5	6	7
2. Emotion (unchanging facial expression, blank stare, expressionless face)	1	2	3	4	5	6	7
3. Reduced social drive	1	2	3	4	5	6	7
4. Poor grooming and hygiene	1	2	3	4	5	6	7

Score:_____

Sources of information (check all applicable):
_____Patient
_____Parents/Relatives
_____Mental health professionals
_____Chart

Explain here if validity of assessment is questionable:
_____ Symptoms possibly drug-induced
_____ Underreported due to lack of rapport
_____ Underreported due to negative symptoms
_____ Patient is uncooperative
_____ Difficult to assess due to formal thought disorder
_____ Other_____

---

[1]Reprinted with permission from Chiles JA, Miller AL, Hall CS, et al.: *Texas Implementation of Medication Algorithms (TIMA): Schizophrenia Module. Administration Manual: 4-Item Positive Symptom Rating Scale and Brief Negative Symptom Assessment*, Version 5.0. Austin, Texas Department of Mental Health and Mental Retardation, 2001.

INSTRUCTIONS FOR USING THE
BRIEF BIPOLAR DISORDER SYMPTOM SCALE (BDSS)

INTRODUCTION

The Brief Bipolar Disorder Symptom Scale (BDSS) is an instrument used by the Texas Implementation of Medication Algorithms (TIMA) in the Texas mental health system for assessing symptoms of bipolar disorder. The BDSS is adapted from the 24-item Brief Psychiatric Rating Scale (Overall and Gorham 1988). The BDSS is divided into three symptom groups: mania/hypomania, major depression, and psychosis. In the mania/hypomania group, five symptoms are scored: hostility, elevated mood, grandiosity, excitement, and motor hyperactivity; in major depression, four symptoms are scored: depressed mood, anxiety, emotional withdrawal, and blunted affect; and in psychosis, only unusual thought content is scored.

BRIEF BIPOLAR DISORDER SYMPTOM SCALE (BDSS)[1]

1. **Hostility:** Animosity, contempt, belligerence, threats, arguments, tantrums, property destruction, fights, and any other expression of hostile attitudes or actions. Do not infer hostility from neurotic defenses, anxiety, or somatic complaints. Do not include incidents of appropriate anger or obvious self-defenses.

How have you been getting along with people (family, co-workers, etc.)?

Have you been irritable or grumpy lately? (How do you show it? Do you keep it to yourself?)

Were you ever so irritable that you would shout at people or start fights or arguments? (Have you found yourself yelling at people you didn't know?)

Have you hit anyone recently?

NA = Not Assessed   **1 = Not Present**

2 = Very Mild: Irritable or grumpy, but not overtly expressed.

3 = Mild: Argumentative or sarcastic.

4 = Moderate: Overtly angry on several occasions OR yelled at others excessively.

5 = Moderately Severe: Has threatened, slammed about or thrown things.

6 = Severe: Has assaulted others but with no harm likely, e.g., slapped or pushed, OR destroyed property, e.g., knocked over furniture, broken windows.

7 = Extremely Severe: Has attacked others with definite possibility of harming them or with actual harm, e.g., assault with hammer or weapon.

---

[1]Reprinted with permission from Suppes T, Dennehy EB: *TIMA Procedural Manual: Bipolar Disorders Algorithms.* Austin, Texas Medication Algorithm Project, Texas Department of Mental Health and Mental Retardation, 2002, pp. 37–48.

2. **Elevated Mood:** A pervasive, sustained, and exaggerated feeling of well-being, cheerfulness, euphoria (implying a pathological mood), optimism that is out of proportion to the circumstances. Do not infer elation from increased activity or from grandiose statements.

Have you felt so good or high that other people thought that you were not your normal self? Have you been feeling cheerful and "on top of the world" without any reason?

[If patient reports elevated mood/euphoria, ask the following:]

Did it seem like more than just feeling good? How long did that last?

NA = Not Assessed   **1 = Not Present**

2 = Very Mild: Seems to be very happy, cheerful without much reason.

3 = Mild: Some unaccountable feelings of well-being that persist.

4 = Moderate: Reports excessive or unrealistic feelings of well-being, cheerfulness, confidence, or optimism inappropriate to circumstances, some of the time. May frequently joke, smile, be giddy, or overly enthusiastic OR few instances of marked elevated mood with euphoria.

5 = Moderately Severe: Reports excessive or unrealistic feelings of well-being, confidence, or optimism inappropriate to circumstances much of the time. May describe "feeling on top of the world," "like everything is falling into place," or "better than ever before" OR several instances of marked elevated mood with euphoria.

6 = Severe: Reports many instances of marked elevated mood with euphoria OR mood definitely elevated almost constantly throughout interview and inappropriate to content.

7 = Extremely Severe: Reports being elated or appears almost intoxicated, laughing, joking, giggling, constantly euphoric, feeling invulnerable, all inappropriate to immediate circumstances.

3. **Grandiosity:** Exaggerated self-opinion, self-enhancing conviction of special abilities or powers or identity as someone rich or famous. Rate only patient's statements about himself, not his demeanor. *Note:* If the subject rates a "6" or "7" due to grandiose delusions, you must rate Unusual Thought Content at least a "4" or above.

Is there anything special about you? Do you have any special abilities or powers? Have you thought that you might be somebody rich or famous?

[If the patient reports any grandiose ideas/delusions, ask the following:]

How often have you been thinking about [use patient's description]*? Have you told anyone about what you have been thinking? Have you acted on any of these ideas?*

NA = Not Assessed   **1 = Not Present**

2 = Very Mild: Feels great and denies obvious problems, but not unrealistic.

3 = Mild: Exaggerated self-opinion beyond abilities and training.

4 = Moderate: Inappropriate boastfulness; claims to be brilliant, insightful, or gifted beyond realistic proportions, but rarely self-discloses or acts on these inflated self-concepts. Does not claim that grandiose accomplishments have actually occurred.

5 = Moderately Severe: Same as 4 but often self-discloses and acts on these grandiose ideas. May have doubts about the reality of the grandiose ideas. Not delusional.

6 = Severe: Delusional—claims to have special powers like ESP, to have millions of dollars, invented new machines, worked at jobs when it is known that he has never been employed in these capacities, be Jesus Christ or the President. Patient may not be very preoccupied.

7 = Extremely Severe: Delusional—same as 6 but subject seems very preoccupied and tends to disclose or act on grandiose delusions.

4. **Depression:** Includes sadness, unhappiness, anhedonia, and preoccupation with depressing topics (cannot attend to TV, conversations due to depression), hopelessness, loss of self-esteem (dissatisfied or disgusted with self or feelings of worthlessness). Do not include vegetative symptoms, e.g., motor retardation, early waking, or the amotivation that accompanies the deficit syndrome.

    How has your mood been recently? Have you felt depressed (sad, down, unhappy as if you didn't care)? Are you able to switch your attention to more pleasant topics when you want to?

    Do you find that you have lost interest in or get less pleasure from things you used to enjoy, like family, friends, hobbies, watching TV, eating?

    [If subject reports *feelings* of depression, ask the following:]

    How long do these feelings last? Has it interfered with your ability to perform your usual activities or work?

    NA = Not Assessed   1 = Not Present

    2 = Very Mild: Occasionally feels sad, unhappy, or depressed.

    3 = Mild: Frequently feels sad or unhappy, but can readily turn attention to other things.

    4 = Moderate: Frequent periods of feeling very sad, unhappy, moderately depressed, but able to function with extra effort.

    5 = Moderately Severe: Frequently, but not daily, periods of deep depression OR some areas of functioning are disrupted by depression.

    6 = Severe: Deeply depressed daily but not persisting throughout the day OR many areas of functioning are disrupted by depression.

    7 = Extremely Severe: Deeply depressed daily OR most areas of functioning are disrupted by depression.

5. **Anxiety:** Reported apprehension, tension, fear, panic, or worry. Rate only the patient's statements, not observed anxiety that is rated under Tension.

    Have you been worried a lot during [mention time frame]? *Have you been nervous or apprehensive? (What do you worry about?)*

    Are you concerned about anything? How about finances or the future?

    When you are feeling nervous, do your palms sweat or does your heart beat fast (or shortness of breath, trembling, choking)?

[If patient reports anxiety or autonomic accompaniment, ask the following:]

How much of the time have you been [use patient's description]*?*

Has it interfered with your ability to perform your usual activities or work?

NA = Not Assessed   **1 = Not Present**

2 = Very Mild: Reports some discomfort due to worry OR infrequent worries that occur more than usual for most normal individuals.

3 = Mild: Worried frequently but can readily turn attention to other things.

4 = Moderate: Worried most of the time and cannot turn attention to other things easily but no impairment in functioning OR occasional anxiety with autonomic accompaniment but no impairment in functioning.

5 = Moderately Severe: Frequent, but not daily, periods of anxiety with autonomic accompaniment OR some areas of functioning are disrupted by anxiety or worry.

6 = Severe: Anxiety with autonomic accompaniment daily but not persisting throughout the day OR many areas of functioning are disrupted by anxiety or constant worry.

7 = Extremely Severe: Anxiety with autonomic accompaniment persisting throughout the day OR most areas of functioning are disrupted by anxiety or constant worry.

6. **Unusual Thought Content:** Unusual, odd, strange, or bizarre thought content. Rate the degree of unusualness, not the degree of disorganization of speech. Delusions are patently absurd, clearly false, or bizarre ideas that are expressed with full conviction. Consider the patient to have full conviction if he/she has acted as though the delusional beliefs were true. Ideas of reference/persecution can be differentiated from delusions in that ideas are expressed with much doubt and contain more elements of reality. Include thought insertion, withdrawal, and broadcast. Include grandiose, somatic, and persecutory delusions even if rated elsewhere. *Note:* If Somatic Concern, Guilt, Suspiciousness, or Grandiosity are rated "6" or "7" due to delusions, the Unusual Thought Content must be rated a "4" or above.

Have you been receiving any special messages from people or from the way things are arranged around you? Have you seen any references to yourself on TV or in the newspaper?

Can anyone read your mind?

Do you have a special relationship with God?

Is anything like electricity, X-rays, or radio waves affecting you?

Are thoughts put into your head that are not your own?

Have you felt that you were under the control of another person or force?

[If patient reports any odd ideas/delusions, ask the following:]

How often do you think about [use patient's descriptions]*?*

Have you told anyone about these experiences? How do you explain the things that have been happening [specify]*?*

NA = Not Assessed   **1 = Not Present**

2 = Very Mild: Ideas of reference (people may stare or may laugh at him), ideas of persecution (people may mistrust him). Unusual beliefs in psychic powers, spirits, UFOs, or unrealistic beliefs in one's own abilities. Not strongly held. Some doubt.

3 = Mild: Same as 2, but degree of reality distortion is more severe as indicated by highly unusual ideas or greater conviction. Content may be typical of delusions (even bizarre), but without full conviction. The delusion does not seem to have fully formed, but is considered as one possible explanation for an unusual experience.

4 = Moderate: Delusion present but no preoccupation or functional impairment. May be an encapsulated delusion or firmly endorsed absurd belief about past delusional circumstances.

5 = Moderately Severe: Full delusion(s) present with some preoccupation OR some areas of functioning disrupted by delusional thinking.

6 = Severe: Full delusion(s) present with much preoccupation OR many areas of functioning are disrupted by delusional thinking.

7 = Extremely Severe: Full delusions present with almost total preoccupation OR most areas of functioning are disrupted by delusional thinking.

7. **Excitement:** Heightened emotional tone, or increased emotional reactivity to interviewer or topics being discussed, as evidenced by increased intensity of facial expressions, voice tone, expressive gestures, or increase in speech quantity and speed.

NA = Not Assessed   **1 = Not Present**

2 = Very Mild: Subtle and fleeting or questionable increase in emotional intensity. For example, at times, seems keyed-up or overly alert.

3 = Mild: Subtle but persistent increase in emotional intensity. For example, lively use of gestures and variation in voice tone.

4 = Moderate: Definite but occasional increase in emotional intensity. For example, reacts to interviewer or topics that are discussed with noticeable emotional intensity. Some pressured speech.

5 = Moderately Severe: Definite and persistent increase in emotional intensity. For example, reacts to many stimuli, whether relevant or not, with considerable emotional intensity. Frequent pressured speech.

6 = Severe: Marked increase in emotional intensity. For example, reacts to most stimuli with inappropriate emotional intensity. Has difficulty setting down or staying on task. Often restless, impulsive, or speech is often pressured.

7 = Extremely Severe: Marked and persistent increase in emotional intensity. Reacts to all stimuli with inappropriate intensity, impulsiveness. Cannot settle down or stay on task. Very restless and impulsive most of the time. Constant pressured speech.

8. **Motor Hyperactivity:** Increase in energy level evidenced in more frequent movement and/or rapid speech. Do not rate if restlessness is due to akathisia.

NA = Not Assessed   **1 = Not Present**

2 = Very Mild: Some restlessness, difficulty sitting still, lively facial expressions, or somewhat talkative.

3 = Mild: Occasionally very restless, definite increase in motor activity, lively gestures, 1–3 brief instances of pressured speech.

4 = Moderate: Very restless, fidgety, excessive facial expressions or nonproductive and repetitious motor movement. Much pressured speech, up to one-third of the interview.

5 = Moderately Severe: Frequently restless, fidgety. Many instances of excessive nonproductive and repetitious motor movements. On the move most of the time. Frequent pressured speech, difficult to interrupt. Rises on 1–2 occasions to pace.

6 = Severe: Excessive motor activity, restlessness, fidgety, loud tapping, noisy, etc., throughout most of the interview. Speech can only be interrupted with much effort. Rises on 3–4 occasions to pace.

7 = Extremely Severe: Constant excessive motor activity throughout entire interview, e.g., constant pacing, constant pressured speech with no pauses, interviewee can only be interrupted briefly and only small amounts of relevant information can be obtained.

9. **Emotional Withdrawal:** Deficiency in patient's ability to relate emotionally during interview situation. Use your own feeling as to the presence of an "invisible barrier" between patient and interviewer. Include withdrawal apparently due to psychotic processes.

NA = Not Assessed   1 = Not Present

2 = Very Mild: Lack of emotional involvement shown by occasional failure to make reciprocal comments, occasionally appearing preoccupied, or smiling in a stilted manner, but spontaneously engages the interviewer most of the time.

3 = Mild: Lack of emotional involvement shown by noticeable failure to make reciprocal comments, appearing preoccupied, or lacking in warmth, but responds to interviewer when approached.

4 = Moderate: Emotional contact not present much of the interview because subject doesn't elaborate responses, fails to make eye contact, doesn't seem to care if interviewer is listening, or may be preoccupied with psychotic material.

5 = Moderately Severe: Same as "4," but emotional contact not present most of the interview.

6 = Severe: Actively avoids emotional participation. Frequently unresponsive or responds with yes/no answers (not solely due to persecutory delusions). Responds with only minimal affect.

7 = Extremely Severe: Consistently avoids emotional participation. Unresponsive or responds with yes/no answers (not solely due to persecutory delusions). May leave during interview or just not respond at all.

10. **Blunted Affect:** Restricted range in emotional expressiveness of face, voice, and gestures. Marked indifference or flatness even when discussing distressing topics. In the case of euphoric or dysphoric patients, rate Blunted Affect if a flat quality is also clearly present.

Use the following probes at end of interview to assess emotional responsivity:

Have you heard any good jokes lately? Would you like to hear a joke?

NA = Not Assessed   1 = Not Present

2 = Very Mild: Emotional range is slightly subdued or reserved, but displays appropriate facial expressions and tone of voice that are within normal limits.

3 = Mild: Emotional range overall is diminished, subdued, or reserved, without many spontaneous and appropriate emotional responses. Voice tone is slightly monotonous.

4 = Moderate: Emotional range is noticeably diminished; patient does not show emotion, smile, or react to distressing topics except infrequently. Voice tone is monotonous or there is noticeable decrease in spontaneous movements. Displays of emotion or gestures are usually followed by a return to flattened affect.

5 = Moderately Severe: Emotional range very diminished; patient doesn't show emotion, smile, or react to distressing topics except minimally; few gestures, facial expression does not change very often. Voice tone is monotonous much of the time.

6 = Severe: Very little emotional range or expression. Mechanical in speech and gestures most of the time. Unchanging facial expression. Voice tone is monotonous most of the time.

7 = Extremely Severe: Virtually no emotional range or expressiveness, stiff movements. Voice tone is monotonous all of the time.

Sources of information (check all applicable):

_____ **Patient**

_____ **Parents/Relative**

_____ **Mental health professional**

_____ **Chart**

Explain here if validity of assessment is questionable:

_____ **Symptoms possibly drug-induced**

_____ **Underreported due to lack of rapport**

_____ **Underreported due to negative symptoms**

_____ **Patient uncooperative**

_____ **Difficult to assess due to formal thought disorder**

_____ **Other reason_____**

Confidence in assessment:

_____ **1 (= not at all) through 5 (= very confident)**

REFERENCES

Overall JE, Gorham DR: The Brief Psychiatric Rating Scale (BPRS): recent developments in ascertainment and scaling. Psychopharmacol Bull 24:97–99, 1988

Suppes T, Dennehy EB: TIMA Procedural Manual: Bipolar Disorders Algorithms. Austin, Texas Medication Algorithm Project, Texas Department of Mental Health and Mental Retardation, 2002, pp 37–48

Brief Bipolar Disorder Symptom Scale (BDSS)[1]

Symptom group	Symptoms	NA	1	2	3	4	5	6	7
Manic / Hypomanic	Hostility								
	Elevated mood								
	Grandiosity								
	Excitement								
	Motor hyperactivity								
Major depressive	Depressed mood								
	Anxiety								
	Emotional withdrawal								
	Blunted affect								
Psychotic	Unusual thought content								

Patient: _____   **Date:** _____

Instructions: Indicate the score for each item in the appropriate cell to the right of the item. Evaluate the pattern and severity of symptom(s) to guide clinical decision making.

NA = Not Assessed   1 = Not Present   2 = Very Mild   3 = Mild   4 = Moderate   5 = Moderately Severe   6 = Severe   7 = Extremely Severe

Scale Total: _____

[1]Reprinted with permission from Suppes T, Dennehy EB: *TIMA Procedural Manual: Bipolar Disorders Algorithms.* Austin, Texas Medication Algorithm Project, Texas Department of Mental Health and Mental Retardation, 2002, pp. 37–48.

INSTRUCTIONS FOR USING THE HAMILTON RATING SCALE FOR DEPRESSION (HAM-D)

DESCRIPTION

The Hamilton Rating Scale for Depression (Ham-D) (Hamilton 1960) is one of the most widely used instruments for the clinical assessment of depression. The scale was developed in 1960 and has been well validated since. It remains the standard against which other depressive scales are evaluated.

The Ham-D has 17–21 items, depending on the version used. The original scale had 21 items, and Hamilton suggested scoring only the first 17 items because the last 4 items either occurred infrequently (e.g., depersonalization) or did not measure the severity of the illness (e.g., diurnal variation) (American Psychiatric Association 2000). Most clinicians and treatment studies of depression use the 17-item version. Regardless of the version, the Ham-D is a scale for assessing the severity of depression for patients with a diagnosis of primary depressive disorder. The scale emphasizes the somatic symptoms of depression that are sensitive to change. Thus, Ham-D can be an invaluable instrument to assess the efficacy of antidepressant therapy.

ADMINISTRATION OF THE HAM-D

A physician or a trained rater should administer the Ham-D. The scale does not have standardized questions but relies on the skills of the interviewer to collect and evaluate the information in making rating decisions. It takes approximately 30 minutes to administer the scale. The rater evaluates the severity of the symptoms on the basis of the information gained from questions that concentrate on the patient's condition during the last few weeks or days. Additional information from relatives, friends, nurses, and others who are familiar with the patient may be taken into consideration in weighing the score.

A modified version of the Ham-D, and the one that is widely used, was published in the Early Clinical Drug Evaluation Program (ECDEU) (Guy 1976). Symptoms on this scale are rated finely (on a 5-point scale) and coarsely (on a 3-point scale). Scores on the 5-point scale are equivalent to the following: 0 = absent; 1 = doubtful or trivial; 2 = mild; 3 = moderate; and 4 = severe. Scores on the 3-point scale are equivalent to the following: 0 = absent; 1 = doubtful or mild; and 3 = obvious, distinct, or severe.

In one published report (Kerns et al. 1982), the scores on the Ham-D were compared with scores on other scales that measured symptom severity of depression. The following thresholds were derived for Ham-D scores: very severe, >23; severe, 19–22; moderate, 14–18; mild, 8–13; and normal, ≤7.

REFERENCES

American Psychiatric Association: Handbook of Psychiatric Measures. Washington, DC, American Psychiatric Association, 2000

Guy W: ECDEU Assessment Manual for Psychopharmacology, Revised Edition (DHEW Publ No ADM 76-388). Washington, DC, U.S. Dept of Health, Education and Welfare, 1976

Hamilton M: A rating scale for depression. J Neurol Neurosurg Psychiatry 23:56–64, 1960

Kerns NP, Cruickshank CA, McGuigan KJ, et al: A comparison of depression rating scales. Br J Psychiatry 141:45–49, 1982

HAMILTON RATING SCALE FOR DEPRESSION (HAM-D)[1]

Patient's name: _____ Date of this interview: _____

Chart no.: _____ D.O.B.: _____ Date of last interview: _____

Physician or rater: _____

Current therapy: _____

_____

1. Depressed Mood   *Feelings of sadness, hopelessness, helplessness, worthlessness*

☐   0 = Absent
☐   1 = These feeling states indicated only on questioning.
☐   2 = These feeling states spontaneously reported verbally.
☐   3 = Communicates feeling states nonverbally, i.e., through facial expression, postures, voice, and tendency to weep
☐   4 = Patient reports *virtually only* these feeling states in his spontaneous verbal and non-verbal communication

2. Feelings of Guilt

☐   0 = Absent
☐   1 = Self-reproach, feels he has let people down
☐   2 = Ideas of guilt or rumination over past errors or sinful deeds
☐   3 = Present illness is a punishment. Delusions of guilt.
☐   4 = Hears an accusatory or denunciatory voices and/or experiences threatening visual hallucinations

3. Suicide

☐   0 = Absent
☐   1 = Feels life is not worth living
☐   2 = Wishes he were dead or any thoughts of possible death to self
☐   3 = Suicide ideas or gestures
☐   4 = Attempts at suicide (*any serious attempt rates 4*)

4. Insomnia Early

☐   0 = No difficulty falling asleep
☐   1 = Complains of occasional difficulty falling asleep—i.e., more than ½ hour
☐   2 = Complains of nightly difficulty falling asleep

5. Insomnia Middle

☐   0 = No difficulty
☐   1 = Patient complains of being restless and disturbed during the night
☐   2 = Waking during the night—any getting out of bed rates 2 (*except for purpose of voiding*)

6. Insomnia Late

☐   0 = No difficulty
☐   1 = Waking in early hours of the morning but goes back to sleep
☐   2 = Unable to fall asleep if gets out of bed

_____

[1]Reprinted from Hamilton M: "A Rating Scale for Depression." *Journal of Neurology, Neurosurgery, and Psychiatry* 23:56–64, 1960.

7. Work and Activities

- ☐ 0 = No difficulty
- ☐ 1 = Thoughts and feelings of incapacity, fatigue, or weakness related to activities, work, or hobbies
- ☐ 2 = Loss of interest in activity, hobbies, or work—either directly reported by patient, or indirect in listlessness, indecision, and vacillation *(feels he has to push self to work or activities)*
- ☐ 3 = Decrease in actual time spent in activities or decrease in productivity. In hospital, rate 3 if patient does not spend at least three hours a day in activities *(hospital job or hobbies)*, exclusive of ward chores.
- ☐ 4 = Stopped working because of present illness. In hospital, rate 4 if patient engages in no activities except ward chores, or if patient fails to perform ward chores unassisted.

8. Retardation   *Slowness of thought and speech, impaired ability to concentrate, decreased motor activity*

- ☐ 0 = Normal speech and thought
- ☐ 1 = Slight retardation at interview
- ☐ 2 = Obvious retardation at interview
- ☐ 3 = Interview difficult
- ☐ 4 = Complete stupor

9. Agitation

- ☐ 0 = None
- ☐ 1 = "Playing with" hands, hair, etc.
- ☐ 2 = Hand-wringing, nail-biting, hair-pulling, biting of lips

10. Anxiety Psychic

- ☐ 0 = No difficulty
- ☐ 1 = Subjective tension and irritability
- ☐ 2 = Worry about minor matters
- ☐ 3 = Apprehensive attitude apparent in face or speech
- ☐ 4 = Fears expressed without questioning

11. Anxiety Somatic   *Physiological concomitants of anxiety, such as:*

- ☐ 0 = Absent   *Gastrointestinal—dry mouth, wind, indigestion, diarrhea, cramps, belching*
- ☐ 1 = Mild   *Cardiovascular—palpitations, headaches*
- ☐ 2 = Moderate   *Respiratory—hyperventilation, sighing*
- ☐ 3 = Severe   *Urinary frequency*
- ☐ 4 = Incapacitating *Sweating*

12. Somatic Symptoms Gastrointestinal

- ☐ 0 = None
- ☐ 1 = Loss of appetite, but eating without staff encouragement. Heavy feelings in abdomen
- ☐ 2 = Difficulty eating without staff urging. Requests or requires laxatives or medication for bowels or medications for GI symptoms

13. Somatic Symptoms General

- ☐ 0 = None
- ☐ 1 = Heaviness in limbs, back, or head. Backaches, headache, muscle aches. Loss of energy and fatigability
- ☐ 2 = Any clear-cut symptoms rates 2

14. Genital Symptoms   *Symptoms such as loss of libido, menstrual disturbances*

- ☐ 0 = Absent
- ☐ 1 = Mild
- ☐ 2 = Severe

15. Hypochondriasis

- ☐   0 = Not present
- ☐   1 = Self-absorption (bodily)
- ☐   2 = Preoccupation with health
- ☐   3 = Frequent complaints, requests for help, etc.
- ☐   4 = Hypochondriacal delusion

16. Loss of Weight   *(Answer only A or B)*

A. When rating by history:

- ☐   0 = No weight loss
- ☐   1 = Probable weight loss associated with present illness
- ☐   2 = Definite (according to patient) weight loss

B. On weekly ratings by ward psychiatrist, when actual weight changes are measured:

- ☐   0 = Less than 1 lb weight loss in week
- ☐   1 = Greater than 1 lb weight loss in week
- ☐   2 = Greater than 2 lb weight loss in week

17. Insight

- ☐   0 = Acknowledges being depressed and ill
- ☐   1 = Acknowledges illness, but attributes cause to bad food, climate, overwork, virus, need to rest, etc.
- ☐   2 = Denies being ill at all

Total Score on This Interview: _____

Total Score on Previous Interview: _____

INSTRUCTIONS FOR USING THE QUICK INVENTORY OF DEPRESSIVE SYMPTOMATOLOGY (SELF-REPORT) (QIDS-SR)[1]

INTRODUCTION

The QIDS-SR is an abbreviated version of the **Inventory of Depressive Symptomatology (Self-Report)** (IDS-SR; Rush et al. 1996) used in the Texas Medication Algorithm Project (TMAP) for the implementation of the algorithms in the Texas public mental health system. The implementation phase, or Phase 4, of TMAP is also known as the Texas Implementation of Medication Algorithms (TIMA). The IDS-SR was designed as a patient self-reporting instrument to measure signs and symptoms of depression, including all items for major depressive disorder. The IDS-SR is available in a 28- and 30-item version and a clinician-administered instrument (IDS-C). The QIDS-SR, on the other hand, consists of 16 items taken from the IDS-SR and requires less than 15–20 minutes for the patient to complete.

USING THE QIDS-SR

The QIDS-SR consists of 16 individual items that the patient is asked to read and rate based upon his/her individual perception of the presence and severity of common depression-related symptoms. If the patient has difficulty reading or interpreting an item, it is appropriate for a staff member to read the question to the patient, but the staff should not lead or influence the patient's answer. Although some patients may have difficulty using the form for the first time, most individuals should be able to easily complete it after the second or third time. Most patients also appreciate the opportunity to be able to tell the physician and other staff about the symptoms that are bothering them. The QIDS-SR is constructed in order to capture a range of DSM-IV-related depressive symptoms in an individual patient, while minimizing the tendency to overrate selected symptoms (e.g., sleep disturbance). For this reason, the patient does not answer all of the questions. For example, on questions 6 and 7, addressing appetite disturbance, the patient answers only one of the questions (addressing either decreased or increased appetite). If the patient has no appetite disturbance, she/he can answer either question. The same principles apply to questions 8 and 9. The QIDS-SR is also available in Spanish, and this version should be used for individuals who primarily read Spanish.

In scoring the QIDS-SR, the clinician does NOT sum all of the items to get the rating score. The scoring instructions are listed on page 2 of the form. If the form is scored correctly, only 12 of the questions will be summed in obtaining the patient's depression rating score, with a maximum possible score of 27. The scoring criteria for severity of depressive symptoms are listed below. Please note that these scoring criteria are a guideline, and they should never be used as a substitute for the clinician's judgment regarding the clinical status of the patient. Rather they are intended as a tool for the clinician to use in quantifying the severity of depressive symptoms and the response to treatment.

---

[1]Reprinted with permission from Trivedi MH, Shon S, Crismon ML, et al.: "Texas Implementation of Medication Algorithms (TIMA): Guidelines for Treating Major Depressive Disorder," in *TIMA Physician Procedural Manual.* Austin, Texas Medication Algorithm Project, Texas Department of Mental Health and Mental Retardation, Revised September 2000, pp. 62–63.

QIDS-SR Scoring Criteria

Normal	**≤5**
Mild	**6–10**
Moderate	**11–15**
Moderate to Severe	**16–20**
Severe	**≥21**

REFERENCES

Rush AJ, Gullion BM, Basco MR, et al: The Inventory of Depressive Symptomatology (IDS): psychometric properties. Psychol Med 26:477–486, 1996

The QIDS-SR is adapted from the Inventory of Depressive Symptomatology (Self-Report) (IDS-SR), by A. John Rush, M.D., et al.

Trivedi MH, Shon S, Crismon ML, et al: Texas Implementation of Medication Algorithms (TIMA): guidelines for treating major depressive disorder, in TIMA Physician Procedural Manual. Austin, Texas Medication Algorithm Project, Texas Department of Mental Health and Mental Retardation, Revised September 2000, pp 62–63

QUICK INVENTORY OF DEPRESSIVE SYMPTOMATOLOGY (SELF-REPORT) (QIDS-SR)[1]

Name: _____ Date: _____

Please circle the one response to each item that best describes you for the past 7 days.

1. Falling Asleep:

0	I never take longer than 30 minutes to fall asleep.
1	I take at least 30 minutes to fall asleep, less than half the time.
2	I take at least 30 minutes to fall asleep, more than half the time.
3	I take more than 60 minutes to fall asleep, more than half the time.

2. Sleep During the Night:

0	I do not wake up at night.
1	I have a restless, light sleep with a few brief awakenings each night.
2	I wake up at least once a night, but I go back to sleep easily.
3	I awaken more than once a night and stay awake for 20 minutes or more, more than half the time.

3. Waking Up Too Early:

0	Most of the time, I awaken no more than 30 minutes before I need to get up.
1	More than half the time, I awaken more than 30 minutes before I need to get up.
2	I almost always awaken at least 1 hour or so before I need to, but I go back to sleep eventually.
3	I awaken at least 1 hour before I need to and can't go back to sleep.

4. Sleeping Too Much:

0	I sleep no longer than 7–8 hours per night, without napping during the day.
1	I sleep no longer than 10 hours in a 24-hour period, including naps.
2	I sleep no longer than 12 hours in a 24-hour period, including naps.
3	I sleep longer than 12 hours in a 24-hour period, including naps.

5. Feeling Sad:

0	I do not feel sad.
1	I feel sad less than half the time
2	I feel sad more than half the time.
3	I feel sad nearly all of the time.

---

[1]Reprinted with permission from Trivedi MH, Shon S, Crismon ML, et al.: "Texas Implementation of Medication Algorithms (TIMA): Guidelines for Treating Major Depressive Disorder," in *TIMA Physician Procedural Manual.* Austin, Texas Medication Algorithm Project, Texas Department of Mental Health and Mental Retardation, Revised September 2000, pp. 62–63.

Please complete *either* 6 *or* 7, but not both.

6. Decreased Appetite:

0   There is no change in my usual appetite.
1   I eat somewhat less often or lesser amounts of food than usual.
2   I eat much less than usual and only with personal effort.
3   I rarely eat within a 24-hour period, and only with extreme personal effort or when others persuade me to eat.

7. Increased Appetite:

0   There is no change from my usual appetite.
1   I feel a need to eat more frequently than usual.
2   I regularly eat more often and/or greater amounts of food than usual.
3   I feel driven to overeat both at mealtime and between meals.

Please complete *either* 8 *or* 9, but not both.

8. Decreased Weight (within the last 2 weeks):

0   I have not had a change in my weight.
1   I feel as if I've had a slight weight loss.
2   I have lost 2 pounds or more.
3   I have lost 5 pounds or more.

9. Increased Weight (within the last 2 weeks):

0   I have not had a change in my weight.
1   I feel as if I've had a slight weight gain.
2   I have gained 2 pounds or more.
3   I have gained 5 pounds or more.

10. Concentration/Decision Making:

0   There is no change in my usual capacity to concentrate or make decisions.
1   I occasionally feel indecisive or find that my attention wanders.
2   Most of the time, I struggle to focus my attention or to make decisions.
3   I cannot concentrate well enough to read or cannot make even minor decisions.

11. View of Myself:

0   I see myself as equally worthwhile and deserving as other people.
1   I am more self-blaming than usual.
2   I largely believe that I cause problems for others.
3   I think almost constantly about major and minor defects in myself.

12. Thoughts of Death or Suicide:

0   I do not think of suicide or death.
1   I feel that life is empty or wonder if it's worth living.
2   I think of suicide or death several times a week for several minutes.
3   I think of suicide or death several times a day in some detail, or I have made specific plans for suicide or have actually tried to take my life.

13. General Interest:

    0   There is no change from usual in how interested I am in other people or activities.

    1   I notice that I am less interested in people or activities.

    2   I find I have interest in only one or two of my formerly pursued activities.

    3   I have virtually no interest in formerly pursued activities.

14. Energy Level:

    0   There is no change in my usual level of energy.

    1   I get tired more easily than usual.

    2   I have to make a big effort to start or finish my usual daily activities (e.g., shopping, homework, cooking or going to work).

    3   I really cannot carry out most of my usual daily activities because I just don't have the energy.

15. Feeling Slowed Down:

    0   I think, speak, and move at my usual rate of speed.

    1   I find that my thinking is slowed down or my voice sounds dull or flat.

    2   It takes me several seconds to respond to most questions, and I'm sure my thinking is slowed.

    3   I am often unable to respond to questions without extreme effort.

16. Feeling Restless:

    0   I do not feel restless,

    1   I'm often fidgety, wringing my hands, or need to shift how I am sitting.

    2   I have impulses to move about and am quite restless.

    3   At times, I am unable to stay seated and need to pace around.

To Score:

1.   Enter the highest score on any one of the four sleep items (1–4)   _____

2.   Item 5   _____

3.   Enter the highest score on any one appetite/weight item (6–9)   _____

4.   Item 10   _____

5.   Item 11   _____

6.   Item 12   _____

7.   Item 13   _____

8.   Item 14   _____

9.   Enter the highest score on either of the two psychomotor items (15 and 16)   _____

TOTAL SCORE (Range 0–27)   _____

Interpretation of Score

Normal	≤5
Mild	6–10
Moderate	11–15
Moderate to Severe	16–20
Severe	≥21

REFERENCES

Rush AJ, Gullion BM, Basco MR, et al: The Inventory of Depressive Symptomatology (IDS): psychometric properties. Psychol Med 26:477–486, 1996

The QIDS-SR is adapted from the Inventory of Depressive Symptomatology (Self-Report) (IDS-SR), by A. John Rush, M.D., et al.

Trivedi MH, Shon S, Crismon ML, et al: Texas Implementation of Medication Algorithms (TIMA): guidelines for treating major depressive disorder, in TIMA Physician Procedural Manual. Austin, Texas Medication Algorithm Project, Texas Department of Mental Health and Mental Retardation, Revised September 2000, pp 62–63

Instructions for Using the
Mini-Mental State Examination (MMSE)

The Mini-Mental State Examination (MMSE) of Folstein et al. (1975) is a widely used screening test for measuring cognitive impairment in the elderly, but it can be used with many kinds of patients when there might be cognitive impairment. It takes about 5 minutes to complete when used by itself and adds about 2–3 minutes when it is embedded into the Mental Status Examination section of the *Initial Psychiatric History and Assessment* (Form 1–8). It measures orientation to time and place, registration of information (immediate recall; can information get in and out of the brain?), attention and calculation, short-term memory, language, and construction ability. It is easy to use and score. It can be adapted to almost any clinical situation as long as the patient is cooperative.

Although a normal range for the general population has not been established, most cognitively healthy people will score close to the maximum score of 30. Items on which normal individuals will often make mistakes are recalling the three objects (most normal individuals will remember at least one or two objects). Some individuals, depending on their educational background, will have difficulty subtracting serial 7s to 65. Individuals who read little may have some difficulty remembering the proper order of the less recent presidents. Others may have difficulty copying the interlocking five-sided figure correctly. Occasionally, an otherwise healthy individual simply cannot perform this task. However, a change in performance on the construction task is usually important.

In Folstein et al.'s (1975) original publication, a group of 63 normally functioning individuals with an average age of 74 years had a mean score of 27.6 and a range of 24 to 30. Because intelligence, educational background, and cultural background will affect performance, unless there are longitudinal data of a patient's performance on the MMSE, or it can be determined from achievements how a patient should do (this is much easier when the patient and examiner have the same social and cultural background), the MMSE is not a sensitive screen for early dementia. This is especially true when a patient's psychiatric illness affects his or her performance. However, a patient who does poorly, who is not psychotic or depressed, and who at a previous time was intellectually active very likely has a dementing illness. It should be noted that dementia is not synonymous with irreversibility. At least 20% of dementias are reversible and are caused by drug toxicity, metabolic disorders such as hypothyroidism, or depression.

After a clinician has given the MMSE to enough patients, he or she should gain a fairly clear notion of whether an MMSE examination result is abnormal. Additionally, he or she will know the kinds of errors found in individuals whose apparent cognitive deficits are caused by anxiety or depression or are related to a different cultural or educational background. Generally, patients with dementia will perform worse than patients with depression or schizophrenia, although early during the course of dementia there may be only small deficits. The MMSE should be used as a screening test when there is a question about the cognitive state of an individual. It should be followed up with an appropriate evaluation. The specificity of the MMSE is increased when there are positive release signs, gait disturbances, and impaired stereognosis.

To use the MMSE, try to make the patient comfortable. Try not to hurry; give the patient time to answer the questions and perform the tasks. Although there is some evidence that there is greater reliability when the MMSE is timed, many clinicians find they obtain more valid results if the patient is allowed to produce his or her best results, and a little extra time may encourage this outcome in a confused patient. On the other hand, allowing a patient to dwell on mistakes may breed anxiety and more errors. It is therefore important that the approach be encouraging and positive, even when a patient does poorly. Statements such as "good try" for failures and praise for success are usually welcome.

The patient should be made to feel comfortable and the examination given after there has been an opportunity to establish rapport, without the pressure of time.

REFERENCES

Folstein MF, Folstein SE, McHugh PR: Mini-Mental State: a practical method for grading the cognitive state of patients for the clinician. J Psychiatr Res 12:189–198, 1975

MINI-MENTAL STATE EXAMINATION (MMSE)[1]

Patient's name: _____   **Date:** _____

Orientation	Score 1 for each correct (Max = 10)	
Where are you? *(Ask general, then specific questions to the right.)*	Name this place (building or hospital).	
	What floor are you on now?	
	What state are you in?	
	What county are you in? (If not in a county, score correct if city is correct.)	
	What city are you in (or near) now?	
What is the date today? *(Ask general, then specific questions to the right.)*	What year is it?	
	What season is it?	
	What month is it?	
	What is the day of the week?	
	What is the date today?	
Registration	Score 1 for each object correctly repeated (Max = 3)	
	Name three objects (ball, flag, and tree) and have patient repeat them. (If patient misses object, ask patient to repeat them after you until he or she learns them. Stop at 6 repeats.)	(Say objects at about 1 word per second.)	
Attention and Calculation	Score 1 for each correct to 65 (Max = 5)	
	Subtract 7s backwards from 100 in a serial fashion to 65. Alternatively, ask serial 3s from 20 or spell *WORLD* backwards.		
Recall	Score 1 for each object recalled (Max = 3)	
	Do you recall the names of the three objects?		
Language		
	Ask patient to provide names of a watch and pen as you show them to him.	Score 1 for each object correct (Max = 2)	
	Repeat "No ifs, ands, or buts" (only one trial).	Score 1 if correct	
	Give patient a piece of plain blank paper and say, "Take the paper in your right hand (1), fold it in half (2), and put it on the floor (3)."	Score 1 for each part done correctly (Max = 3)	
	Ask patient to read and perform task written on paper: "Close your eyes."	Score 1 if patient closes eyes	
	Ask patient to write a sentence on a piece of paper.	Score total of 1 if sentence has a subject, object, and verb (Max = 1)	
Construction		
	Ask patient to copy the design of the interlocking five-sided figures.	Score total of 1 if all 10 angles are present and 2 angles intersect; ignore tremor and rotation (Max = 1)	
Total score	(Maximum score = 30)	

---

[1]Adapted with permission from Folstein MF, Folstein SE, McHugh PR: "Mini-Mental State: A Practical Method for Grading the Cognitive State of Patients for the Clinician." *Journal of Psychiatric Research* 12:189–198, 1975.

INSTRUCTIONS FOR USING THE YALE-BROWN OBSESSIVE COMPULSIVE SCALE (Y-BOCS)

The Yale-Brown Obsessive Compulsive Scale (Y-BOCS) of Goodman et al. (1989) is not used to make a diagnosis, but to assess the severity of the symptoms of obsessive-compulsive disorder (OCD) and to follow response to treatment. Intensity of symptoms, subjective distress, control, resistance, and interference are rated for the previous 7 days. Interference of activities is the impairment of social and occupational function. Feelings of resistance indicate the patient's effort in countering obsessional thinking and compulsive behavior.

To be able to determine changes over time and maintain consistency, symptoms are to be rated for the last week, not for a specific time and not specifically on the day of testing. The Y-BOCS is divided into two sections: obsessive and compulsive. The scores for each section range from 0 to 20. When scores for the two sections of the Y-BOCS are added, a total score of 25 or more is considered moderately severe, a score of 30 or more is considered severe, and a score of more than 35 is considered very severe.

I have found that it takes a considerable amount of time to feel comfortable using the Y-BOCS. For many patients, estimating the time spent thinking about an obsession or a compulsion is a difficult task. It is much easier to use on an inpatient unit or when significant others can be asked for input. Otherwise, both patient and rater must work together over time to learn to make consistent ratings.

Generally the Y-BOCS is more sensitive to changes in obsessive-compulsive symptoms than to symptoms of anxiety and depression, although at times they will seem to go hand in hand. The scale might also be used when patients with psychotic disorders improve. It is not uncommon for them to become more obsessive and at times compulsive. For some patients, this result is a way of ordering what has been a disorderly life; for others, it may be a medication side effect, such as occurs with higher doses of clozapine.

REFERENCES

Goodman WK, Price LH, Rasmussen SA, et al: The Yale-Brown Obsessive Compulsive Scale, I: development, use, and reliability. Arch Gen Psychiatry 46:1006–1011, 1989

YALE-BROWN OBSESSIVE COMPULSIVE SCALE (Y-BOCS)

Patient's name: _____   **Date:** _____

Item		None	Mild	Moderate	Severe	Extreme
1. Hours/day spent on obsessions		0	0 to 1	>1 to 3	>3 to 8	>8
	Score	0	1	2	3	4
2. Interference from obsessions		None	Mild	Definite but manageable	Impaired	Incapacitating
	Score	0	1	2	3	4
3. Distress from obsessions		None	Mild	Moderate but manageable	Severe	Near constant, disabling
	Score	0	1	2	3	4
4. Resistance to obsessions		Always resists	Much resistance	Some resistance	Often yields	Completely yields
	Score	0	1	2	3	4
5. Control over obsessions		Complete control	Much control	Moderate control	Little control	No control
	Score	0	1	2	3	4
					Obsession Subscale (0–20)	
6. Hours/day spent on compulsions		0	0 to 1	>1 to 3	>3 to 8	>8
	Score	0	1	2	3	4
7. Interference from compulsions		None	Mild	Definite but manageable	Impaired	Incapacitating
	Score	0	1	2	3	4
8. Distress from compulsions		None	Mild	Moderate but manageable	Severe	Near constant, disabling
	Score	0	1	2	3	4
9. Resistance to compulsions		Always resists	Much resistance	Some resistance	Often yields	Completely yields
	Score	0	1	2	3	4
10. Control over compulsions		Complete control	Much control	Moderate control	Little control	No control
	Score	0	1	2	3	4
					Compulsion Subscale (0–20)	
					Total Score (0–40)	

Comments:

Date: _____

Total previous score: _____

Range of severity: 0–7 Subclinical; 8–15 Mild; 16–23 Moderate; 24–31 Severe; 32–40 Extreme. Ratings include observations during interviews as well as average occurrence for each item during the last 7 days.

Source Adapted with permission from Goodman WK, Price LH, Rasmussen SA, et al.: "The Yale-Brown Obsessive Compulsive Scale, I: Development, Use, and Reliability." *Archives of General Psychiatry* 46:1006–1011, 1989.

INSTRUCTIONS FOR USING THE
ABNORMAL INVOLUNTARY MOVEMENT SCALE (AIMS)

The AIMS is a standardized, widely used aid for the examination and recording of abnormal involuntary movements (National Institute of Mental Health 1975). Ideally, it is used before the administration of neuroleptics and regularly thereafter.

The AIMS Is Not a Diagnosis

The AIMS is a method for monitoring the presence of abnormal movements; by itself it cannot make the diagnosis of tardive dyskinesia. Diagnosing tardive dyskinesia requires using criteria described elsewhere (Baldessarini et al. 1980; Jeste and Wyatt 1982; Jeste et al. 1984; Kane et al. 1992; Schooler and Kane 1982).

Examination Procedure for the AIMS

The standardized procedure for performing the AIMS, described below, has been extensively used by epidemiologists and other researchers. Although standardization of the procedure is important for many reasons, deviation from the protocol is common in clinical practice.

The chair to be used in this examination should be hard, firm, and without arms. Very good discussions on how to perform the AIMS can be found in articles by Munetz and Benjamin (1988) and Lane et al. (1985).

1. Ask the patient if there is anything in his or her mouth (i.e., gum, candy, etc.), and if there is, ask him or her to please remove it.

2. Ask the patient about the condition of his or her teeth. Ask the patient if he or she wears dentures. Are the patient's teeth or dentures bothering him or her?

3. Ask the patient whether he or she has noticed any movements around or in his or her mouth, face, hands, or feet. If "yes," ask the patient to describe them and to what extent they are a bother or interfere with his or her activities. *(Comment:* Besides asking about choreiform and choreoathetoid movements, this is a good time to ask about akathisia. Ask the patient if he or she feels the need to move his or her feet or other parts of the body. Ask the patient if he or she feels jittery, anxious, restless, or like jumping out of his or her skin. Ask the patient if his or her mind feels fuzzy or if he or she is having difficulty focusing [cognitive akathisia]. Questions relating to akathisia probably should be asked much more often than the formal AIMS usually is performed.)

4. Have the patient sit on a chair with hands on knees, legs slightly apart, and feet flat on the floor. Look at entire body for movements while in this position. *(Comment:* This is a good time to look at respiratory movements; be sure to look for diaphragm movements. When the patient talks, note any laryngeal or pharyngeal dyskinesias.)

5. Ask the patient to sit with hands hanging unsupported—if male, between his legs, and if female and wearing a dress, hands over her knees. Observe hands and other body areas. *(Comment:* The point here is to keep the hands and fingers unsupported.)

6. Ask the patient to open his or her mouth. Observe the tongue at rest within the mouth. Do this twice.

7. Ask the patient to protrude his or her tongue from his or her mouth ("Stick your tongue out!"). Observe abnormalities of tongue movement. Do this twice. (*Comment:* Can the patient keep his or her tongue protruded outside his mouth? If the patient forgets to keep the tongue out, it is likely to be related to inattention. If the tongue goes in and out of the mouth, the movements might be choreoathetoid and related to tardive dyskinesia.)

8. Ask the patient to tap his or her thumb to each finger on the same hand sequentially, as rapidly as possible for 10–15 seconds. Do this separately with the right hand, then with the left hand. Observe facial and leg movements. *(Comment:* This is the *first activation movement.* On activation, score only choreiform and choreoathetoid movements. Do not score normal-appearing movements of the opposite side of the body or tongue protrusion if it is not accompanied by choreic movements. Such movements are usually "overflow" movements and may be normal or part of another neurological condition. Watch the patient's legs for restlessness [e.g., shaking the leg from the knee]. Do not score restlessness as dyskinesia; it may be related to anxiety or akathisia.)

9. Passively flex and extend the patient's left and right arms at the shoulder, elbow, and wrist (one at a time). Note any rigidity. (*Comment:* Do not confuse rigidity with dystonia, which may be part of tardive dyskinesia or tardive dystonia. Rigidity is not part of tardive dyskinesia but may mask dyskinesias. In addition to neuroleptic-induced parkinsonism and Parkinson's disease, lithium, some frontal lobe syndromes, Alzheimer's disease, other dementias, and pyramidal and extrapyramidal tract disorders can produce cogwheeling and other forms of rigidity.)

10. Ask the patient to stand up. Observe in profile. Observe all body areas again, hips included. (*Comment:* Be sure to look at the patient from the front, sides, and back. If the patient has akathisia—while standing it might be seen as marching in place—score it separately from dyskinetic movements.)

11. Ask the patient to extend his or her arms with the palms down. Look for tremors. Observe trunk, legs, and mouth. (*Comment:* This is the *second activation movement.* Do not focus only on the extended arms. Look at the whole body, including the toes.)

12. Have the patient walk a few paces, turn, and walk back to the chair. Observe hands and gait. Do this twice. (*Comment:* This is the *third activation movement.* The arms, hands, and fingers may be placed into odd dystonic movements, which are not necessarily part of tardive dyskinesia or tardive dystonia. Such dystonias may be related to lesions of the extrapyramidal system, and often are called mannerisms.)

Scoring Procedure

Complete the examination procedure before making rating.

For the movement ratings (the first three categories below), rate the highest severity observed.

0 = none; 1 = minimal (may be extreme normal); 2 = mild; 3 = moderate; 4 = severe; NR = not ratable. According to the original AIMS instructions, one point is subtracted if movements are seen only on activation, but not all investigators follow that convention.

Facial and Oral Movements

1. **Muscles of facial expression**

   Rate movements of the forehead, eyebrows, and periorbital area, including blinking and frowning (do not rate lower facial areas here). (Estimating the blink rate is optional. The suggestions for scoring the blink rate are far from exact and if used should serve as very rough guidelines. Some patients with abnormal facial-expression movements will show no change in, or a decrease in, blink rate. To estimate the blink rate, use a hand-held counter and only count blinks when patient is quiet and not talking.)

Minimal: Rare frowns unrelated to apparent emotion being expressed occur once every 2–3 minutes (or blink rate is slightly elevated [i.e., 20–25 per minute]).

Mild: Forehead and periorbital movements of mild intensity occur every 1–2 minutes (or blink rate is greater than 25 per minute).

Moderate: Forehead and periorbital movements of moderate amplitude occur several times per minute (or blink rate is greater than 30 per minute).

Severe: Forehead and periorbital movements of large amplitude occur several or more times per minute (or blink rate is greater than 40 per minute).

2. Lips and perioral region

Rate the degree to which cheeks puff out and lips pucker, pout, or smack together. (Do not rate a lip movement if it is secondary to tongue or jaw movements. Secondary movements are passive movements. If the upper and lower lips move simultaneously, they are probably not secondary and should be rated here.)

Minimal: Movements occur only 2–3 times during 5 minutes of observation and may be an exaggeration of normal facial expression.

Mild: Movements occur once every 1–2 minutes and are clearly abnormal.

Moderate: Abnormal movements of marked amplitude occur several times per minute or more often if the amplitude is mild.

Severe: Abnormal movements occur several times per minute and are of marked amplitude.

3. Jaw

Rate the severity of biting, clenching, chewing, mouth opening, and lateral movements.

Minimal: Movements occur only several times in 5 minutes with an amplitude that is on the upper limits of normal (i.e., less than 50% of the estimated maximum amplitude or muscle strength).

Mild: Movements of approximately 50% maximum strength/amplitude occur every 1–3 minutes.

Moderate: Movements of approximately 50% maximum strength/amplitude occur 3–6 times per minute or movements that are greater than 50% maximum strength/amplitude occur every 1–3 minutes.

Severe: Movements of at least 50% maximum strength/amplitude occur fairly continuously or movements of close to 100% of maximum strength/amplitude occur every 10–20 seconds.

4. Tongue

Examine the tongue in the following three situations: a) Observe the tongue during the general examination. If it moves laterally within the mouth and/or in and out of the mouth, rate the movement. b) Ask the patient to open his or her mouth and observe the tongue. The anchor points described below are for the tongue during this period. 3) Ask the patient to stick out his or her tongue twice. If the patient cannot or will not open his or her mouth, rate tongue movements by observing the larynx with the patient's mouth closed.

Minimal: Tongue may go partly in or out, but not fully so, or it may wander from midline (no more than twice) but not reach the teeth.

Mild: Tongue goes in or out 1–3 times or wanders from midline and touches the teeth 1–3 times.

Moderate: Tongue moves more than 3 times but not continually. It must go past the teeth.

Severe: Tongue moves continuously in and out, past the teeth, or laterally.

Extremity Movements

5. Upper Extremities

Rate the patient's arms, wrists, hands, or fingers for choreic (rapid, jerky, irregular, purposeless) or athetotic (slow, sinuous, purposeless) movements.

Minimal: Movements of small amplitude occur several times within a 5-minute period.

Mild: Movements of small to moderate amplitude occur several times within a 2-minute period.

Moderate: Fairly continuous movements of small amplitude are observed or movements of moderate amplitude occur several times within a 30-second period.

Severe: Continuous movements of at least moderate amplitude are present.

6. Lower Extremities

Examine legs, knees, ankles, and toes for choreic or athetotic movements. Also include lateral knee movements, foot squirming and tapping, heel dropping, and inversion/eversion of foot. Use the same criteria for upper extremities as instructed in item 5.

Trunk Movements

7. Trunk

Rate neck, shoulders, and hips for twisting, rocking, and gyrating movements. Rate for presumed choreoathetoid movements based on breathing patterns, vocalizations, and any observed abdominal and chest wall movements.

Minimal:	Movements of small amplitude occur only several times in 5 minutes.
Mild:	Movements of small amplitude occur several times per minute.
Moderate:	Movements of medium amplitude seen every 12–20 seconds.
Severe:	Movements of medium amplitude that are fairly continuous or movements of high amplitude seen every 20–30 seconds are observed. Considerable dystonia is often present.

Global Judgments

8. **Severity of abnormal movements based on the highest single score items.**

9. **Incapacitation due to abnormal movements.**

10. **Patient's awareness of abnormal movements.**

Dental Status

11. **Current problems with teeth and/or dentures?**   0 = No; 1 = Yes

12. **Does patient usually wear dentures?**   0 = No; 1 = Yes

REFERENCES

Baldessarini RJ, Cole JO, Davis JM, et al: Tardive Dyskinesia: A Task Force Report of the American Psychiatric Association. Washington, DC, American Psychiatric Association, 1980

Egan MF, Hyde TM, Albers GW, et al: Treatment of tardive dyskinesia with vitamin E. Am J Psychiatry 149:773–777, 1992

Jeste DV, Wyatt RJ: Understanding and Treating Tardive Dyskinesia. New York, Guilford, 1982

Jeste DV, Karson CN, Wyatt RJ: Movement disorders and psychopathology, in Neuropsychiatric Movement Disorders. Edited by Jeste DV, Wyatt RJ. Washington, DC, American Psychiatric Press, 1984, pp 119–150

Kane JM, Jeste DV, Barnes TRE, et al: Tardive Dyskinesia: A Task Force Report of the American Psychiatric Association. Washington, DC, American Psychiatric Association, 1992

Lane RD, Glazer WM, Hansen TE, et al: Assessment of tardive dyskinesia using the Abnormal Involuntary Movement Scale. J Nerv Ment Dis 173:353–357, 1985

Munetz MR, Benjamin S: How to examine patients using the Abnormal Involuntary Movement Scale. Hosp Community Psychiatry 39:1172–1177, 1988

National Institute of Mental Health, Psychopharmacology Research Branch: Abnormal Involuntary Movement Scale. Early Clinical Drug Evaluation Unit Intercomunication 4:3–6, 1975

Schooler HR, Kane JM: Research diagnoses for tardive dyskinesia. Arch Gen Psychiatry 39:486–487, 1982

ABNORMAL INVOLUNTARY MOVEMENT SCALE (AIMS)

Symptoms	Month / Date / Year			
	/ /	/ /	/ /	/ /
Facial and Oral Movements	(circle one)	(circle one)	(circle one)	(circle one)
1. **Muscles of facial expressions** (e.g., movements of forehead, eyebrows, periorbital area, cheeks; include frowning, blinking, smiling, grimacing)	0 1 2 3 4 NR	0 1 2 3 4 NR	0 1 2 3 4 NR	0 1 2 3 4 NR
2. **Lips and perioral area** (e.g., puckering, pouting, smacking)	0 1 2 3 4 NR	0 1 2 3 4 NR	0 1 2 3 4 NR	0 1 2 3 4 NR
3. **Jaw** (e.g., biting, clenching, chewing, mouth opening, lateral movement)	0 1 2 3 4 NR	0 1 2 3 4 NR	0 1 2 3 4 NR	0 1 2 3 4 NR
4. **Tongue** Rate only movements both in and out of mouth. NOT inability to sustain movement.	0 1 2 3 4 NR	0 1 2 3 4 NR	0 1 2 3 4 NR	0 1 2 3 4 NR
Extremity Movements				
5. **Upper extremities (arm, wrist, hand, fingers)** Include choreic movements (i.e., rapid, objectively purposeless, irregular, spontaneous), athetoid movements (i.e., slow irregular, complex, serpentine). Do not include tremor (i.e., repetitive, regular, rhythmic).	0 1 2 3 4 NR	0 1 2 3 4 NR	0 1 2 3 4 NR	0 1 2 3 4 NR
6. **Lower extremities (legs, wrists, hands, fingers)** (e.g., lateral knee movements, foot tapping, heel dropping, food squirming, inversion and eversion of foot)	0 1 2 3 4 NR	0 1 2 3 4 NR	0 1 2 3 4 NR	0 1 2 3 4 NR
Trunk Movements				
7. **Neck, shoulders, hips** (e.g. rocking twisting, squirming, pelvic gyrations)	0 1 2 3 4 NR	0 1 2 3 4 NR	0 1 2 3 4 NR	0 1 2 3 4 NR
Global Judgments				
8. **Severity of abnormal movements**	0 1 2 3 4 NR	0 1 2 3 4 NR	0 1 2 3 4 NR	0 1 2 3 4 NR
9. **Incapacitation due to abnormal movements**	0 1 2 3 4 NR	0 1 2 3 4 NR	0 1 2 3 4 NR	0 1 2 3 4 NR
10. **Patient's awareness of abnormal movements** Rate only patient's report	0 1 2 3 4 NR	0 1 2 3 4 NR	0 1 2 3 4 NR	0 1 2 3 4 NR
Miscellaneous	<u>Yes</u>	<u>No</u>		
11. **Current problems with teeth and/or dentures?**			If "yes", what kind?	
12. **Dentures present?**				
13. **Has patient's score changed significantly since last time?**				
14. **If yes, has the patient been informed?**				

Rate the highest severity observed. Rate movements that occur upon activation 1 less than those observed spontaneously.

Code: 0 = None; 1 = Minimal; 2 = Mild; 3 = Moderate; 4 = Severe; NR = Not Ratable

Part 2: Information About Psychiatric Illnesses for Patients and Families

INFORMATION ABOUT

ALZHEIMER'S DISEASE

FOR PATIENTS AND FAMILIES

Alzheimer's disease is the most common and well-known form of degenerative **dementia**. By definition, dementia is a **syndrome**, a cluster of symptoms, of impaired memory and cognition. Dementia is a **cognitive disorder** that impairs an individual's memory and ability for reasoning, awareness, and judgment. Cognitive impairment in Alzheimer's disease may involve disturbance of language (**aphasia**), loss of ability to carry out complex motor activities (**apraxia**), and loss of ability to recognize or identify familiar people or objects (**agnosia**). Another common manifestation of Alzheimer's disease is the disturbance of **executive functioning**, which is the ability to initiate, plan, assess, and carry out complex tasks in a logical sequence of steps. The abilities to plan a shopping list, drive to the store, and shop for the items are examples of skills requiring executive functioning.

Alzheimer's disease affects approximately 2.5 million Americans and accounts for 50%–60% of all cases of dementia. It affects less than 1% of people at age 65 in the United States, but the rate doubles approximately every 5 years to 2% at age 70 and 4% at age 75, and by the age of 90 the rate is over 20%. As the segment of population older than 65 years is rapidly increasing in the United States, managing Alzheimer's disease will present a major public health challenge.

COURSE OF ILLNESS

Alzheimer's disease, like many other types of dementia, has an insidious onset. An early manifestation of the disease is memory impairment, which is often overlooked and attributed to aging. As cognitive symptoms appear, the individual may undergo dramatic lifestyle changes. A person who was once active may show loss of motivation and energy, complaining of fatigue and lassitude, which is often diagnosed as depression. Memory disturbance is usually the earliest obvious sign that something is wrong. This may be perilous for the elderly person, who may, for example, forget to turn off the stove or leave the car engine running. Usually, the diagnosis of Alzheimer's disease is not made until the individual develops behavioral symptoms and is brought to the attention of a physician. Behavioral problems may include temper outbursts, daytime wandering, poor hygiene, suspiciousness, making accusations, and physical violence.

The disease as a general rule follows a progressive course of declining cognitive function and memory loss. For some patients, and particularly for those who benefit from medications, the progressive deterioration may stabilize for several years, with a plateau in overall functional impairment, before the progression of the disease continues and cognitive functioning declines further. In the advanced stages of Alzheimer's disease, impairment may be so profound that the patient may no longer be able to recognize family members or perform the most basic tasks of self-feeding and personal hygiene. The patient may become incontinent, hostile with extreme emotional outbursts, and assaultive. Hallucinations and delusions are not uncommon in advanced stages of cognitive deterioration. The management of the patient often takes a heavy toll on the caretakers. From the time symptoms are recognized and a diagnosis is made, the degenerative course of Alzheimer's disease may continue for years until death ensues. The mean survival for patients of Alzheimer's disease is about 10 years but may range from 1 to 20 years.

CAUSE OR ETIOLOGY

The definitive diagnosis of Alzheimer's disease is made at postmortem examination of the patient's brain, from microscopic findings that are hallmarks of the disease. These findings include **neurofibrillary tangles**, which are formed when a type of protein found in neurons (brain cells) is defective. The defective protein twists in "tangles" and becomes ineffective in carrying out normal cellular functions. Ultimately, this leads to cell death and Alzheimer's disease.

Another important finding is **amyloid plaques**. Amyloid plaques are derived from the aberrant formation of a neuronal protein. The resultant abnormal protein makes up the core of amyloid plaques. How these plaques result in cellular damage and destruction is unclear. One explanation is that plaques cause cellular inflammation and damage. The abnormal deposit of amyloid plaques may be analogous to cholesterol deposits and plaque formation along arterial walls, causing arteriosclerosis and arterial damage. Ultimately, the destruction of brain cells is the final pathway leading to the cause Alzheimer's disease.

Recent advances in genetic mapping provide compelling evidence that the formation of tangles and plaques in Alzheimer's disease may be genetically linked. Alzheimer's disease may be due to mutations (i.e., random changes in the genetic material) on particular chromosomes (i.e., the DNA in our genes). One explanation is that the neurons with the abnormal gene result in the production of an altered protein that causes formation of amyloid deposits that leads to Alzheimer's disease. Another explanation is that an amyloid transport protein, which binds and transports amyloid from the brain, is abnormal and therefore ineffective in removing amyloid. The amyloid transporting protein is called **apolipoprotein E** (ApoE). Several genes that code for ApoE are associated with the risk of developing late-onset Alzheimer's disease, the most common type of Alzheimer's disease. One of the genes for ApoE is found on **chromosome 19** and is linked to late-onset Alzheimer's disease.

DIAGNOSIS

The diagnosis of Alzheimer's disease is made on the basis of exclusion of other forms of dementia. The initial workup by the physician is to establish that the dementia is not caused by another medical condition. For example, some elderly patients with depressive illness may present with **pseudodementia** with clinical features similar to dementia, including memory and cognitive impairment, but generally the symptoms of pseudodementia are not as severe as those of true dementia. The important distinction is that pseudodementia resolves when the depression is successfully treated. Another important differentiation is to exclude **delirium**, which can also cause disturbance in cognition and may be misdiagnosed as dementia. Once the diagnosis of dementia is made, clinical history, neurological and psychological testing, and laboratory tests will help the physician differentiate Alzheimer's disease from another form of dementia.

For the diagnosis of Alzheimer's disease to be made, the patient's symptoms must meet the diagnostic criteria for dementia of Alzheimer's disease. The diagnosis must include symptoms in two major areas: 1) memory impairment, showing loss of ability to learn new information or to recall previously learned information; and 2) disturbance in one or more areas of cognition, including aphasia, apraxia, agnosia, and executive functioning. The cognitive deficits also cause significant impairment in social and occupational functioning, showing a continuous decline.

Physicians commonly use the **Mini-Mental State Examination** (MMSE) to assess the patient's cognitive functioning. The initial test score is compared with routine testing to evaluate the extent of cognitive decline. It is common for patients with Alzheimer's disease to have a significantly lower score on each subsequent examination.

CLINICAL MANAGEMENT

There is no cure for Alzheimer's dementia. Treatment is aimed at palliating the symptoms of the disease. Management of the disease rests largely on supportive care for the patient, which usually involves the spouse and other family members, taking care of the patient at home until late in the course of the illness when placement in a skilled nursing facility is needed for around-the-clock care.

The treatment of Alzheimer's disease is directed primarily at preserving cognitive functions. The medications for this purpose are known as **cognitive enhancers**. These agents maintain memory and cognitive function but do not alter the course of the disease. As previously discussed, the widespread destruction of neurons is the cause of cognitive deficits in Alzheimer's disease. The neurons involved are predominantly **cholinergic neurons,** which have a role in memory and learning. Cholinergic neurons require **acetylcholine** as the neurotransmitter (i.e., the brain chemical that facilitates transmission of impulses between neurons). Destruction of cholinergic neurons in Alzheimer's disease results in a deficit of this neurotransmitter. Cognitive enhancers increase levels of acetylcholine in the brain, which help to improve memory and other cognitive functions. Patients are more likely to respond to these agents during the early stages of the disease when more cholinergic neurons are intact.

The cognitive enhancers include **tacrine** (Cognex), **donepezil** (Aricept), **rivastigmine** (Exelon), and **galantamine** (Reminyl). These agents exert their action by inhibiting **cholinesterase,** an enzyme that breaks down acetylcholine, to enhance levels of the neurotransmitter. For further discussion of these agents, refer to the handout *Information About Cognitive Enhancers for Patients and Families* (Form 3–28).

Antipsychotic medications may be needed to manage psychotic symptoms associated with late stages of Alzheimer's disease. Psychotic symptoms usually take the form of delusional thinking or nighttime hallucinations. For example, the patient may become assaultive, thinking his or her spouse is an imposter, or the patient may see and talk to imaginary visitors. A low-dose of antipsychotic medications may be prescribed to control agitation, aggression, and assaultiveness. Physicians today are shifting away from prescribing the older, first-generation antipsychotic agents, such as **haloperidol** (Haldol), **fluphenazine** (Prolixin), and **thioridazine** (Mellaril), and are prescribing the newer, second-generation antipsychotic medications, such as **aripiprazole** (Abilify), **olanzapine** (Zyprexa), **quetiapine** (Seroquel), **risperidone** (Risperdal), and **ziprasidone** (Geodon). The second-generation antipsychotics are usually well tolerated compared with the older antipsychotic medications. They are associated with significantly lower incidence of movement disorders known as **extrapyramidal side effects**, such as Parkinson-like symptoms, muscle spasms, and gait disturbance. In general, the lowest effective dose of antipsychotic medication should be used and for the shortest possible duration. Patients with dementia often do not tolerate the central nervous system (CNS) side effects of antipsychotic medications very well.

Other symptoms associated with Alzheimer's disease include depression, anxiety, and other mood disturbances. Mood stabilizers such as **divalproex** (Depakote) may be prescribed to reduce agitation and other mood symptoms. Depressive symptoms occur frequently with Alzheimer's disease. The **selective serotonin reuptake inhibitors** (SSRIs) are generally well tolerated and the preferred antidepressants for patients with dementia. Tricyclic antidepressants, such as **amitriptyline** (Elavil), should be avoided because these agents have significant sedation and anticholinergic (i.e., opposes the action of cholinergic neurons) activity and may further compromise the patient's cognitive function. Anti-anxiety medications are occasionally needed to manage anxiety. The long-acting benzodiazepines, particularly diazepam (Valium) and chlordiazepoxide (Librium), should be avoided in patients with dementia. These agents are slowly eliminated from the body, and the drug and their metabolites may accumulate and could further impair memory and cognition. Because patients with dementia are generally very sensitive to side effects of centrally active medications, psychotropic medications must be used selectively and cautiously in these patients.

If you have any questions about this handout, please consult your physician.

SUPPORT AND ADVOCACY GROUPS

Alzheimer's Association
225 N. Michigan Ave., Floor 17
Chicago, IL 60601-7633
Phone: (312) 335-8700; (800) 272-3900
Fax: (312) 335-1110
E-mail: info@alz.org
Web site: www.alz.org
Supports education, advocacy, and research pertaining to Alzheimer's disease.

INFORMATION ABOUT

ANXIETY DISORDERS

FOR PATIENTS AND FAMILIES

Anxiety disorders are a group of disorders that have different causes but share many symptoms. Anxiety disorders are the most common of the psychiatric illnesses. The core symptoms of anxiety disorders are nervousness, worry, and fear. The patient's symptoms may cause distress and result in some functional impairment. In the spectrum of anxiety disorders, anxieties may be triggered by excessive fear of certain objects or situations (**phobias**), episodes of sudden, inexplicable terror (**panic attacks**), or persistent thoughts and behaviors (**obsessive-compulsive disorder**, or **OCD**). For others, their disorder is characterized by chronic anxiety and worry (**generalized anxiety disorder**, or **GAD**) without a specific identifiable cause like phobic disorder, panic disorder, or OCD. The anxiety disorders include agoraphobia (fear of open space and leaving familiar surroundings), social phobia, generalized anxiety disorder (GAD), panic disorder (with or without agoraphobia), phobic disorders, and OCD. For a discussion of OCD, refer to the handout *Information About Obsessive-Compulsive Disorder (OCD) for Patients and Families* (Form 2–6).

GENERALIZED ANXIETY DISORDER (GAD)

Without the specific symptoms that characterized panic or phobic disorder, generalized anxiety disorder is marked by persistent apprehension, worry, and anxiety that cause distress and result in physical symptoms. People with GAD worry not just some of the time, but incessantly and excessively about life circumstances, including their health, finances, job, family, and potentially hazardous situations (e.g., driving a car). However, persons with GAD do not have episodes of panic attacks typically seen with panic disorders. The usual clinical symptoms of GAD include restlessness or edginess, becoming easily fatigued, difficulty concentrating, irritability, and sleep disturbance. Anxiety may trigger physical symptoms, such as sweating, rapid heartbeat, dry mouth, frequent urination, lightheadedness, and stomach upset. To make the diagnosis of GAD, the physician must eliminate other causes of anxiety, such as substance abuse, medications, medical conditions (e.g. hyperthyroidism), or other psychiatric disorders (e.g., depression).

Generalized anxiety disorder is a relatively common disorder, afflicting approximately 4%–7% of people in the United States. The incidence of GAD may be higher in women, African Americans, and persons under 30 years of age. The treatment for GAD may consist of medications (anti-anxiety agents), psychotherapy, and behavior therapy.

POSTTRAUMATIC STRESS DISORDER (PTSD)

The concept of PTSD was recognized long before the term was introduced in 1980. It was recognized early on that some soldiers suffered from an emotional disorder following the aftermath of war ("shell shock"). Posttraumatic stress disorder, as the diagnosis implies, occurs following a trauma that was either experienced or witnessed by the person. The traumatic experience may leave the person feeling vulnerable, anxious, helpless, depressed, and emotionally numbed. A person may develop PTSD after a physical or sexual assault, experiencing a near-fatal accident or natural disaster, or witnessing violence and death. Following the aftermath of the traumatic experience, the person may continue to develop psychological reactions related to the frightening experience. The essential clinical features of PTSD include having recurrent, intrusive, and distressing recollections of the event, having recurrent distressing dreams of the event (particularly with children), reliving the experience through flashbacks or hallucinations, and developing intense psychological distress and physical symptoms (e.g., sweating, rapid heartbeat) when exposed to cues that trigger recollection of the traumatic event.

The onset of PTSD may begin within hours or days following the traumatic experience, or it may be delayed for months or years. Without treatment the disorder has a chronic course and may last for years. Many patients with PTSD also develop major depression and other anxiety disorders. Furthermore, patients with PTSD are at risk for substance and alcohol abuse.

Clinical management of PTSD involves treating the underlying symptoms with medications and treating the cause of the illness through psychotherapy. The benzodiazepines are the most widely prescribed tranquilizers used for treating anxiety. Depression is a common aftermath of traumatic stress, and an antidepressant medication may be needed to treat depressive symptoms. Antidepressants may help to reduce nightmares and flashbacks and to improve sleep.

Psychotherapy in the form of supportive intervention may be beneficial initially in helping the patient overcome the traumatic experience. Group and family therapy may be helpful in bringing out painful thoughts and emotions, especially guilt, anger, or fear that have been internalized. Other approaches of psychotherapy may involve behavioral techniques for helping the patient overcome phobias or anxiety related to or associated with the traumatic situation. A gradual process of exposing and confronting the patient to the object or situation that evokes the phobia and anxiety may be achieved though desensitization. Another approach is through cognitive-behavior therapy, with which the patient can learn skills to block intrusive thoughts (e.g., flashback) when they occur and learn relaxation and breathing techniques to overcome anxiety.

PANIC DISORDER AND AGORAPHOBIA

Individuals with panic disorder have unexpected, recurrent anxiety (or panic) attacks that trigger a chain of frightening physical reactions. They may be caught totally off guard while engaged in routine activities, when suddenly their heart begins to pound. They have difficulty breathing, feeling as though they are being smothered or choked; they feel lightheaded, dizzy, or faint; they may complain of nausea and abdominal distress. The panic attack leaves them sweating, trembling, and shaking. The initial reaction is that they are having a heart attack and dying. The attacks are sudden, and usually there is no precipitating cause before the onset of a panic attack. Most attacks lasts about 10 minutes. Panic attacks are overwhelmingly frightening, and these patients live in dread of the next attack.

Agoraphobia is a condition in which individuals become frightened when separated from home and family, their source of security. Agoraphobia often accompanies panic disorder.

People with agoraphobia have a fear of leaving home, being in crowded places, or being away from home alone where they cannot suddenly leave if they have a panic attack. They are usually housebound, and they cannot travel any distance alone away from home without feeling anxious and fearful. They are only able to leave their house or travel when accompanied with someone.

Many experts believe that panic disorder and agoraphobia are a single illness rather than separate disorders. A significant number of persons with panic disorder develop some symptoms of agoraphobia. Panic disorder is classified with or without agoraphobia. Individuals with panic disorder may develop agoraphobia because they fear having a panic attack in a public place where they may not be in control of the situation and feel they may embarrass themselves, or being away from home where they cannot seek help. In some cases, agoraphobia may persist even in the absence of a recent panic attack because these individuals are so preoccupied with fears of another panic attack that they are frightened when separated from their secure surroundings.

The cause of panic disorder has been extensively studied. The etiology of the disorder is associated to an area of the brain stem (**locus coeruleus**) that regulates alertness. Disturbance in this area of the brain stem is the most plausible explanation for causing panic attacks. Therefore, panic disorder is a biological rather than a psychological disturbance that underlies the disorder.

Treatment of panic disorder has the greatest success when a combination of medications and psychotherapy is used. Antidepressants, including the **selective serotonin reuptake inhibitors** (SSRIs), **tricyclic antidepressants** (TCAs), and **monoamine oxidase inhibitors** (MAOIs), are effective for treating panic attacks and agoraphobia in up to 80% of patients. The SSRIs and newer antidepressants have essentially replaced the TCAs and MAOIs because they are better tolerated and safer. For a discussion of these antidepressants, refer to the handouts on SSRIs (Form 3–14), TCAs (Form 3–15), and MAOIs (Form 3–12).

Benzodiazepines (e.g., Valium) are also very effective in blocking panic attacks, but higher doses are required than for treating anxiety disorder. The concern with chronic use of benzodiazepines at high doses is the potential for habituation. Benzodiazepines are also effective for treating the anxiety of panic disorder and agoraphobia, for which they may be prescribed in lower doses than for panic attacks.

Propranolol (Inderal), an adrenergic-blocking agent, may be useful in treating panic attacks for some patients, but it is much less effective than antidepressants or benzodiazepines. Panic disorder may be associated with excessive activity of the adrenergic neurotransmitter system (e.g., norepinephrine). Propranolol antagonizes the adrenergic action of the neurotransmitter and attenuates the symptoms of panic attacks. For example, propranolol may diminish palpitations, rapid heartbeat, sweating, trembling or shaking, and chills or hot flashes during a panic attack.

Psychotherapy in the form of cognitive-behavioral therapy has been effective for treating patients with panic disorder, particularly those with agoraphobia. Cognitive-behavioral therapy usually involves the patient with distraction and breathing exercises and teaches him or her to gain control at the onset of distressing symptoms. With such cognitive-behavioral treatment, along with education, the patient can better understand the illness.

PHOBIC DISORDERS

A *phobia* is defined as an irrational, intense, and persistent fear of an object, place, or situation. A person with a phobia will go to great lengths to avoid the object of fear. What separates normal and usual fear from phobias is that phobic fears are irrational and excessive. Phobias are the most common type of anxiety disorders. There are three types of phobias: agoraphobia, social phobia, and specific phobia. Agoraphobia was discussed earlier in this handout.

Individuals with **social phobia** (also called **social anxiety disorder**) are fearful and anxious when they are in situations around other people where they may be observed or embarrassed. As a result, social anxiety disorder interferes and limits social relationships. These individuals commonly avoid public places where there are crowds.

Specific phobias are extreme fears of animals, objects, places, or situations. The most common types of phobias are fear of snakes, insects, closed spaces (claustrophobia), and heights (acrophobia).

Most individuals with phobias do not seek treatment and only do so when the disorder becomes so incapacitating as to disrupt normal function. Most people circumvent their phobias by avoiding the thing they fear. When individuals with social phobia seek medical attention, a combination of medication and behavior therapy has proved to be the most effective treatment. Antidepressants are effective for treating phobic disorders, and the SSRIs are the commonly prescribed antidepressants because they are well tolerated and generally safe.

Behavior therapy is very effective in the treatment of phobic disorders, both social and specific phobias, using the techniques of exposure and desensitization and flooding. Through the technique of exposure and desensitization, patients are gradually exposed to their fearful situations until they become desensitized to their fears. For example, patients with phobia of snakes may be shown pictures of snakes, and as their fears decrease gradually, they may be asked to visit snakes at the zoo. In the technique of flooding, patients are expected to confront their fears by total exposure to the situation. For example, patients with social phobias may be asked to enter into a situation (e.g., engage a conversation with a stranger) and stay with the situation until their anxiety subsides. With each subsequent encounter, their anxiety becomes less intense.

If you have any questions about this handout, please consult your physician.

ADVOCACY AND SUPPORT GROUPS

Anxiety Disorders Association of America
8730 Georgia Avenue, Suite 600
Silver Spring, MD 20910
Phone: (240) 485-1001
Fax: (240) 485-1035
Web site: www.adaa.org

TERRAP (TERRitorial APprehension)
648 Menlo Avenue, Suite 5
Menlo Park, CA 94025
Phone: (415) 327-1312
Web site: www.terrap.org

INFORMATION ABOUT

ATTENTION-DEFICIT/HYPERACTIVITY DISORDER

FOR PATIENTS AND FAMILIES

Attention-deficit/hyperactivity disorder (ADHD) is a common psychiatric disorder in young and school-aged children. However, it is not merely a childhood disorder. In recent years, an increasing number of adults have been diagnosed with ADHD, raising some concern that it may be overdiagnosed. Estimates of the prevalence (i.e., percentage of the population affected) of ADHD in the United States range from 2% to 12%, and the disorder is about three times more likely in boys than in girls. For most children the disorder improves with maturation, but follow-up studies have shown that a significant number of cases of ADHD persist into adulthood.

Children with ADHD are typically inattentive, very distractible, overactive, impulsive, labile, and difficult to manage. During preschool years, early symptoms and behavioral problems may be passed off simply as manifestations of an active, impetuous child. When the child enters school and begins the task of learning, the disorder then becomes more obvious. The child may have difficulty sitting still, staying focused, completing assignments, and obeying classroom rules. The teacher, school nurse, or school psychologist are usually the first to recognize the child's ADHD and inform the parents to seek help for the child.

COURSE OF DISORDER

Generally, ADHD is not diagnosed before 5 years of age because of the difficulty of differentiating the disorder from the normal developmental stages of toddlers when hyperactivity may be the norm. The period of "terrible twos," for example, is a normal phase of childhood rather than an exception. ADHD is usually not identified until elementary school, when the child is placed in a routine structured environment where attentiveness and sitting still are instilled. In this environment, the child may stand out in comparison to his or her peers.

The outcome of ADHD is variable. According to experts, children with ADHD frequently have good outcome and outgrow the disorder with maturation. However, approximately 50% of childhood ADHD persists with attention deficit and impulsivity into adulthood. The hyperactivity usually improves by early adolescence, but mild symptoms of restlessness and fidgeting may still be seen in some adults. Adults with ADHD may continue to show inattention, impulsivity, and emotional lability without prominent features of hyperactivity.

Treatment also influences outcome. Long-term studies have documented the improvement of children treated with stimulants, especially when compared with children who did not receive medications. Clinical improvement was seen in attention, impulsivity, hyperactivity, and emotional lability. Attenuation of these symptoms helped "normalize" children during critical stages of learning and social development. Moreover, with behavioral improvement, children were likely to receive less negative criticism and more positive reinforcement from parents, teachers, peers, and siblings to improve their self-esteem. The long-term studies also found that children who were treated with stimulants and then followed into adolescence and adulthood had completed more years of school, had fewer automobile accidents, had fewer problems with alcohol and substance abuse, and engaged in less criminal behavior and had fewer court appearances. Therefore, when the natural course of ADHD is changed and improved with treatment, the secondary complications from low self-esteem, compromised social skills, and behavioral problems may be prevented.

CAUSE OR ETIOLOGY

Studies show that ADHD runs in families, particularly in male relatives of ADHD children, but it is unclear how the disorder is transmitted. There is no evidence that ADHD is caused by a single, identifiable genetic defect. Genetic transmission of ADHD will probably be explained by a group of genes that controls or modifies the inheritance of the disorder.

There are nongenetic explanations of ADHD, as well. Recognized nongenetic causes of ADHD include brain damage, low birth weight, and prenatal factors, including inadequate maternal nutrition, alcohol, and substance abuse. Brain damage may result from obstetrical complications, viral infections, and exposure to toxins. Low birth weight is correlated with ADHD, with or without birth complications. In some cases, low birth weight may be attributed to lack of prenatal care (e.g., malnutrition) and substance abuse. Fetal exposure to toxic substances, including alcohol and lead, may predispose to ADHD and cognitive deficits. For example, **fetal alcohol syndrome** includes hyperactivity, attention deficit, and impulsivity, as well as other physical problems.

The manifestation of ADHD may be explained by aberrations of neurotransmitter systems in areas of brain that mediate attention. ADHD may be associated with the neurons (brain cells) that require **dopamine** and **norepinephrine** as their neurotransmitters (i.e., brain chemicals that facilitate transmission of impulses between neurons). Low levels of these neurotransmitters in specific and interrelated areas of the brain that regulate attention, regardless of the cause, may result in the symptoms of attention-deficit and hyperactivity. A depletion of dopamine may result in difficulties in sustaining attention, and depletion of norepinephrine may be responsible for hyperactivity. The most compelling evidence to support this hypothesis is the treatments prescribed for ADHD—medications such as **amphetamine** (Dexedrine) and **methylphenidate** (Ritalin)— work by enhancing the levels of dopamine and norepinephrine.

DIAGNOSIS

The diagnosis of ADHD is based on presentation of symptoms in two broad categories: A) inattention and B) hyperactivity and impulsivity. The diagnostic criteria[1] for ADHD include the following:

A. Symptoms of Inattention

1. Often fails to give close attention to details or makes careless mistakes in schoolwork, work, or other activities

2. Often has difficulty sustaining attention in tasks or play activities

3. Often does not seem to listen when spoken to directly

4. Often does not follow through on instructions and fails to finish schoolwork, chores, or duties (not due to oppositional behavior or failure to understand instructions)

5. Often has difficulty organizing tasks and activities

6. Often avoids, dislikes, or is reluctant to engage in tasks that require sustained mental effort (such as schoolwork or homework)

7. Often loses things necessary for tasks or activities (e.g., toys, school assignments, pencils, books, or tools)

---

[1]Adapted from American Psychiatric Association: *Diagnostic and Statistical Manual of Mental Disorders,* 4th Edition, Text Revision. Washington, DC, American Psychiatric Association, 2000. Copyright 2000, American Psychiatric Association. Used with permission.

8. Is often easily distracted by extraneous stimuli

9. Is often forgetful in daily activities

B. Symptoms of Hyperactivity–Impulsivity

Hyperactivity

1. Often fidgets with hands or feet or squirms in seat

2. Often leaves seat in classroom or in other situations in which remaining seated is expected

3. Often runs about or climbs excessively in situations in which it is inappropriate (in adolescents or adults, may be limited to subjective feelings of restlessness)

4. Often has difficulty playing or engaging in leisure activities quietly

5. Is often "on the go" or often acts as if "driven by a motor"

6. Often talks excessively

Impulsivity

1. Often blurts out answers before questions have been completed

2. Often has difficulty awaiting turn

3. Often interrupts or intrudes on others (e.g., butts into conversations or games)

For the diagnosis of ADHD to be established, the symptoms of inattention and/or hyperactivity-impulsivity must have persisted for at least 6 months. Three subtypes of ADHD are recognized: 1) **Predominantly Hyperactive-Impulsive Type** is the subtype if six (or more) symptoms in the hyperactivity-impulsivity category but fewer than six symptoms in the inattention category are met. 2) **Predominantly Inattentive Type** is the subtype if six (or more) symptoms in the inattention category but fewer than six symptoms in the hyperactivity-impulsivity category are met. This type of ADHD is sometimes referred to as **Attention-Deficit Disorder,** or **ADD.** 3) **Combined Type** is the subtype if six (or more) symptoms in the inattention category and six (or more) symptoms in the hyperactivity-impulsivity category are met. Most children and adolescents with ADHD have the combined type.

Other diagnostic criteria for ADHD include the onset of some symptoms of ADHD before age 7, the symptoms cause dysfunction in at least two settings (e.g., at school and at home), and there is clear evidence that the symptoms affect social or academic functioning.

Because the diagnostic criteria are very explicit in defining a childhood onset, ADHD is not generally diagnosed in adults without a documented childhood history of the disorder. Adults with ADHD usually have problems sustaining attention and controlling impulses but have fewer problems with hyperactivity than do children with ADHD. Unlike childhood ADHD, in which boys are three to four times more likely to have ADHD than girls, men and women are equally prone to the disorder. Therapy for ADHD in kids and adults is essentially the same.

TREATMENT

The primary treatment for ADHD is with medications, and stimulants are medications most commonly prescribed. The benefits of stimulants for treating the core features of ADHD (i.e., hyperactivity, impulsivity, and inattentiveness) are documented by numerous controlled studies and supported by decades of clinical experience. Commonly prescribed stimulants include **methylphenidate** (Ritalin, Metadate, and Concerta),

amphetamine (Dexedrine), **amphetamine mixture** (Adderall), and **pemoline** (Cylert). For a discussion of stimulants used in treatment of ADHD, see the handout *Information About Amphetamines and Methylphenidate for Patients and Families* (Form 3–27).

Nonstimulant medications prescribed for ADHD include antidepressants, **clonidine** (Catapres), **guanfacine** (Tenex), and a recently introduced medication, **atomoxetine** (Strattera). Nonstimulant medications that can enhance levels of dopamine and norepinephrine in the brain may be as effective in treating ADHD as stimulants.

Tricyclic antidepressants (a group of antidepressants that are chemically similar by their three-ring structures) enhance various brain neurotransmitters, including norepinephrine. The tricyclic antidepressants used to treat ADHD with some success include **imipramine** (Tofranil), **desipramine** (Norpramin), and **nortriptyline** (Pamelor).

Nontricyclic antidepressants prescribed for treatment of ADHD include **bupropion** (Wellbutrin) and **venlafaxine** (Effexor).

Clonidine and guanfacine, two medications commonly used for treatment of high blood pressure and other medical conditions, are also effective in treating ADHD. These agents also exert their action in the areas of the brain involved with cognition and attention.

Atomoxetine represents the most recent agent introduced for treating ADHD. It works by blocking the reuptake of norepinephrine back into nerve cells, enhancing neurotransmission of the neurons in areas of the brain involved with cognition and attention. For a discussion of atomoxetine, as well as clonidine and guanfacine, refer to the handout *Information About Nonstimulants for the Treatment of Attention-Deficit/Hyperactivity Disorder for Patients and Families* (Form 3–26).

The treatment of ADHD also emphasizes nonmedical management through behavior modification techniques, involving parents and teachers at home and in school. Behavior modification procedures, for example, emphasize establishing daily checklists for the child, setting limits, providing feedback to the child to reinforce desired behavior, and focusing on success to reinforce self-esteem. Parents learn to become more proactive in managing their child's behavior. They are encouraged to provide a setting that reduces the amount of stimulation for the child and thereby diminish distractibility and inattentiveness. Parents are also encouraged to work closely with their child to tackle tasks in small increments that are best suited to the child's attention span and to reinforce the desired behavior through positive feedback.

If you have questions about this handout, please consult your physician.

ADVOCACY AND SUPPORT GROUPS

Attention Deficit Disorder Association
1788 Second Street, Suite 200
Highland, Park, IL 60035
Phone: (847) 432-2332
Web site: www.add.org

Learning Disabilities Association of America
4156 Library Road
Pittsburgh, PA 15234-1349
Phone: (412) 341-1515
Web site: www.ldanatl.org

Children and Adults Wth Attention-Deficit /
   Hyperactivity Disorder (CHADD)
8181 Professional Place, Suite 150
Landover, MD 20785
Phone: (800) 233-4050; (301) 306-7070
Web site: www.chadd.org

INFORMATION ABOUT

BIPOLAR DISORDER

FOR PATIENTS AND FAMILIES

Bipolar disorder, also called manic-depressive disorder, is a recurrent illness in which the individual's mood cycles between depression and mania with periods of normality. The illness is a *mood disorder*. The individual's moods may swing from manic euphoria, with boundless energy in pursuit of grandiose plans, to depths of depression, with feelings of despair and hopelessness.

During a depressive episode, the patient presents with depressed mood and loss of interest or pleasure. The patient may complain of fatigue, loss of energy almost every day, difficulty sleeping or sleeping too much, diminished ability to concentrate or think, and loss of appetite with significant weight loss. The depressed mood is reported as feelings of sadness, hopelessness, indifference, or worthlessness. Thinking may be slowed, muddled, and confused. The patient often complains of aches and pains, appears tearful, and reveals inappropriate guilt. These symptoms may be accompanied by recurrent thoughts of death or suicide and suicide attempt.

Cycling into a manic episode, the patient's mood may turn abnormally elevated and expansive—inflated with self-confidence or self-importance, euphoria, and exuberance. There is decreased need for sleep. The manic patient typically possesses elevated levels of energy in pursuit of grandiose plans or pleasurable activities. For example, the patient may engage in unrestrained spending sprees, make outrageous business deals, or have heightened sexual drive. Judgment may become severely impaired, resulting in impulsive, uncharacteristic, or inappropriate behavior.

Manic patients generally have rapid thinking, and their speech is rushed or pressured to keep pace with their racing thoughts. They talk excessively, and their speech is marked by a rapid flow of thought or flight of ideas, incoherence, and distractibility. Their mood, at one time euphoric and exuberant, may just as quickly shift, becoming irritable or agitated, especially when they are tired and exhausted from hours without sleep.

In both depressive and manic states of bipolar disorder, patients may manifest psychotic symptoms. However, psychosis is more frequent during manic than depressive states. Psychotic symptoms may include hallucinations and delusions. The content of the hallucinations and delusions is usually consistent with the patient's expansive mood (**mood congruent**). For example, the patient may talk of possessing special powers or abilities, and the delusion would be consistent with the patient's euphoric and grandiose mood. Sometimes the delusions may not be consistent with the mood (**mood incongruent**). For example, the patient may have paranoid delusions of thinking someone is after him or her, although the patient is in a state of euphoria.

There are patients with bipolar disorder who have symptoms of depression and mania simultaneously—that is, a mixture of both depressive and manic symptoms within a single episode. This condition is known as a **mixed state**. In the mixed state, the patient's moods and symptoms are rapidly shifting, at one moment tearfully depressed and suicidal and the next moment engagingly talkative, grandiose, and euphoric.

There is another type of bipolar disorder that presents with manic symptoms that are milder, less severe, and of shorter duration than full-blown mania. This milder form of mania is known as **hypomania**. During a hypomanic episode, patients may experience many of the symptoms of mania but are usually not so impaired as to require hospitalization. Moreover, they do not have hallucinations and delusions. In this type of bipolar disorder, the patient cycles between major depression and hypomania with periods of remission.

Bipolar disorder also exists in a milder condition in which the patient fluctuates between chronic hypomanic and mild depressive states. This type of mood disorder is called **cyclothymia**. During depressive and hypomanic episodes, the patient's symptoms are less severe and incapacitating than during major depression and mania.

COURSE OF ILLNESS

Bipolar disorder usually begins with depression during adolescence. The depression often waxes and wanes until the appearance of the first manic episode. The onset is frequently abrupt but may also occur gradually over the course of several weeks. The prognosis for mania is generally good, especially as treatment has improved with recent medications. Unfortunately, the illness has a significant risk of recurrence, and commonly, after a manic episode the patient cycles into depression. On the other hand, some patients may not experience a full manic episode but exhibit hypomanic states that alternate with depressive episodes.

Generally, untreated individuals have an increased frequency of cycling and longer periods of disability, especially as they get older. In contrast, patients who receive treatment usually do better, with less frequent and severe mood swings. However, there are patients who have an illness marked by **rapid cycling** despite treatment. These patients have at least four episodes of major depressive, manic, hypomanic, or mixed state within 12-month period, and they require closer monitoring and management of their medications.

CAUSE OR ETIOLOGY

The observed patterns of transmission from family studies have provided the best evidence that mood disorders are hereditarily (genetically) linked. In patients with bipolar disorder, family members (particularly among immediate relatives) show a significantly higher rate of mood disorders, especially bipolar disorder, as compared with other psychiatric patients. Approximately 50% of all bipolar disorder patients have at least one parent with a mood disorder, and when both parents have bipolar disorder, there is a 50%–75% chance that a child will have a mood disorder.

Studies of identical and fraternal twins provide even stronger evidence that mood disorders are genetically linked. Data from these studies show that when one identical twin has a mood disorder, there is, on average, a 60% chance that the other sibling will also develop the disorder, whereas in fraternal twins, the rate is only about 5%–25% that the other sibling will develop the disorder.

TREATMENT

Medications are the principal treatment for bipolar disorder. Treatment is directed at treating acute episodes of mania and depression and preventing the recurrence of symptoms after an acute episode. Medications that are used for treating mania are referred to as *mood stabilizers*. This handout shall focus primarily on the treatment of mania. For a discussion on the treatment of depression, refer to the handout *Information About Depressive Disorders for Patients and Families* (Form 2–5). Also, refer to the handouts for discussion of mood stabilizers and antidepressants.

Lithium carbonate is one of the first-line mood stabilizers used in the management of acute mania. It is effective for treatment of acute mania and for prophylaxis to prevent recurrence of mania and depression. Lithium must be dosed cautiously and monitored closely because of its potential for toxicity. Physicians usually prescribe lithium at a dosage of 1,200 to 2,400 mg/day, administered in divided doses, for acute mania. The goal is to attain a blood level of 0.6 to 1.4 mEq per liter. Within this range, the lithium is generally at a therapeutic level, but above the range, lithium toxicity becomes a concern. One of the disadvantages of lithium in treating acute mania is that there is a delay of 5–10 days before patients become fully responsive to the medication.

Another frequently used first-line mood stabilizer for acute mania is valproate, which comes in two different forms: valproic acid and divalproex. The most widely used form is **divalproex** (Depakote). Valproate is also an anticonvulsant that is used for treating and preventing seizures. For mania, divalproex may be given as a single dose or in divided doses in the range of 1,250 to 2,500 milligrams per day. The goal is to achieve therapeutic blood levels in the range of 50 to 125 micrograms per milliliter. Other anticonvulsants used as mood stabilizers for bipolar disorder include **carbamazepine** (Tegretol), **gabapentin** (Neurontin),

lamotrigine (Lamictal), and **oxcarbazepine** (Trileptal). However, these agents are used as alternatives when patients do not respond to lithium or valproate.

During an acute manic episode, the patient may be severely agitated or psychotic. An antipsychotic or benzodiazepine (Valium-like medications) can be administered to control psychotic symptoms and agitation. For example, if the patient is severely psychotic, agitated, or violent and is not cooperating, haloperidol (Haldol), an antipsychotic, and lorazepam (Ativan), a benzodiazepine, may be administered by injections via an intramuscular route. As these symptoms abate, the antipsychotic and benzodiazepine may be gradually discontinued. For some patients with residual psychosis or manic symptoms, continuing the antipsychotic medication may be necessary. Invariably, manic patients will need to be maintained on a mood stabilizer to prevent relapse. To prevent recurrence of depression in bipolar disorder, antidepressants may be added to the medication regimen.

ELECTROCONVULSIVE THERAPY (ECT)

ECT may be a life-saving treatment for severe depression, particularly in patients who at risk for suicide, since it tends to work more quickly than antidepressant medications. Generally, it is indicated when the patient is not responding to medications.

SUPPORTIVE PSYCHOTHERAPY

Supportive psychotherapy may be an invaluable adjunct to medications. A goal of psychotherapy is to identify the external, as well as the internal, issues in the patient's daily life that can exacerbate his or her illness and to devise copying skills to deal with these stressors. Psychotherapy may help the patient deal with the shame, fear, and anxiety of his or her illness. In supportive psychotherapy, the therapist provides the patient with encouragement and directions to cope and overcome difficult situations.

If you have any questions about this handout, please consult your physician.

SUPPORT AND ADVOCACY GROUPS

Lithium Information Center
Madison Institute of Medicine
7617 Mineral Point Road, Suite 300
Madison, WI 53717
Phone: (608) 827-2470
Web site: www.miminc.org/aboutlithinfoctr.html
Provides information on use of lithium for treatment of bipolar disorder and other medical uses.

Depression and Bipolar Support Alliance
  (DBSA)
730 N. Franklin Street, Suite 501
Chicago, IL 60610-3526
(312) 642-0049
(800) 826-3632
www.dbsalliance.org
A patient-directed support alliance that promotes education about depressive and bipolar illnesses.

National Foundation for Depressive Illness, Inc.
P.O. Box 2257
New York, NY 10116
Phone: (800) 239-1265
Web site: www.depression.org
Serves to educate the public about depressive illness and to provide information and referrals to professional help.

National Mental Health Association (NMHA)
2001 N. Beauregard Street, 12th Floor
Alexandria, VA 22311
(703) 684-7722
(800) 969-NMHA
www.nmha.org
A nonprofit organization that serves to promote education and research of mental health and mental illness.

INFORMATION ABOUT

DEPRESSIVE DISORDERS

FOR PATIENTS AND FAMILIES

Depression may simply be transient feelings of dejection and sadness from disappointments, rejections, and losses that are a part of our lives. On the other hand, it may be from grieving the loss of a loved one. These feelings of sadness are usually less severe and are shorter in duration than untreated **major depression** (a more severe form of depression). In milder forms of depression, although psychotherapy and medications may help the individual deal with feelings of sadness and loss, the body's natural recuperative ability eventually "heals the mind."

On the other hand, major depression is a clinical diagnosis of a more severe form of depression. A depressive episode may come on suddenly or insidiously, developing gradually without a precipitating cause. Besides altering mood, major depression also affects bodily functions and thinking. Patients with clinical symptoms of major depression frequently present with changes in sleep, appetite, and daily activity. The depressed patient may have difficulty sleeping or may sleep too much. He or she may have diminished appetite or may eat excessively. There may be significant weight loss without dieting, or weight gain. The patient feels lack of energy and is apathetic, fatigued, or sluggish and leaden. Depression is often associated with somatic (bodily) complaints, with unusual aches and pains, and it is not uncommon for the patient to seek medical attention for what he or she believes are physical ailments, when, in fact, the primary problem may be depression.

Psychologically patients may experience impaired concentration, feelings of guilt, worthlessness, hopelessness, indifference, and loss of interest and ability to feel pleasure (**anhedonia**). Thinking may be slowed, muddled, and confused. Patients often complain of memory problems. They may feel overwhelmed with sadness and express concerns of having a "nervous breakdown." Thoughts of death and suicide are common, and the risk of committing suicide is especially high in depressed patients.

Delusions are false beliefs or perceptions about something or someone. **Hallucinations** are false sensations. These sensations can be heard (auditory), seen (visual), smelled (olfactory), tasted, (gustatory), or felt (tactile).

Delusions and hallucinations may occur in severely depressed patients. The content of the patient's delusions or hallucinations may be consistent with the depression and may be manifested by perceptions of inadequacy, guilt, death, or deserved punishment. Or, the content of the delusions and hallucinations may be more bizarre and may be manifested in symptoms of persecutory delusions (the patient may have delusions in which others want to hurt him), thought insertion (the patient thinks his thoughts are implanted in his mind by other people or forces), and thought broadcasting (the patient thinks her thoughts are broadcasted and can be heard by others). Major depression with delusional or hallucinatory symptoms is a severe form of major depression (**psychotic depression**), requiring aggressive treatment, including use of antipsychotic medications.

Patients with manic-depression, or **bipolar disorder**, may be afflicted with both manic and depressive episodes, with mood swings that take the patient from expansive, manic states to depressive states of hopelessness and despair. The symptoms are almost indistinguishable during a depressive episode in bipolar disorder from major depression.

COURSE OF ILLNESS

The risk of depression extends throughout life. It may begin during any age period, from childhood, adolescence, adulthood, and old age. Generally, depressions are treatable with medications with successful results. However, some patients may not respond to medications, while others may not respond fully and have residual symptoms.

Without treatment, a depressive episode may last for months or even years, but usually it clears spontaneously in about 6 months. However, in patients treated with antidepressants, their depressive episodes last about 3 months (underscoring the importance of antidepressant therapy). Unfortunately, major depression is a chronic disorder, and there is a high rate of relapse. A significant number of patients will have recurrence of their depression. Fortunately, if the patient's first depressive episode was successfully treated, and if it recurs, subsequent depressive episodes will usually respond well to treatment. However, patients who have recurring depressive episodes usually do much better if they continue taking antidepressants. By continuing antidepressants, recurrences are often averted, and if they do occur, they are usually much less severe.

RISK OF SUICIDE

The risk of suicide is very high during the early stages of major depression. Approximately 10%–15% of severely or clinically depressed patients will take their own lives. The risk of suicide is increased in depressed patients who live alone, were recently divorced, have a history of alcohol and drug abuse, have a history of previous suicide attempts, and have expressed suicidal ideations. Patients who are considered high risk for suicide should be hospitalized for inpatient treatment and kept under close watch until they are stabilized.

CAUSE OF DEPRESSION

The study of clinical depression has focused on the neurobiology of the brain and abnormalities in neurotransmission. When earlier studies indicated that antidepressants such as imipramine and monoamine oxidase inhibitors worked by boosting the level of the neurotransmitter **norepinephrine**, scientists postulated that depression might be caused by a deficit of norepinephrine in certain nerve cells throughout the brain. However, with the discovery of fluoxetine (Prozac), another very effective antidepressant, which does not act on the norepinephrine system but instead acts on serotonin, it became evident that other neurotransmitter systems may be involved in depression as well. Understanding depression from a biochemical basis became pivotal to the development of new and improved antidepressants.

Although a biochemical hypothesis to explain the cause of depression may be an oversimplification, it remains useful. It may help patients understand that depression, like other disease processes, is caused by a dysfunction of the body and not a character flaw or weakness. For example, it is analogous to diabetes, in which the disease is caused by low insulin levels or defective insulin regulation and utilization. Similarly, depression may be associated with low levels of neurotransmitters or the abnormal regulation of neurotransmitters. Like many other diseases, depression may be triggered by the environment or inherent in our genes.

Depression may also be caused by a number of physical disorders, the most common of which is decreased thyroid function (hypothyroidism). Occasionally, patients who have strokes become seriously depressed. Depression may occur in women during pregnancy or shortly after childbirth (postpartum depression). Alcohol and drug abuse and certain medications may also cause depression.

DIAGNOSIS

Major Depression

For a diagnosis of major depression, five or more of the following symptoms must be present for at least 2 weeks, and at least one of the symptoms is either depressed mood or loss of interest or pleasure.

- Depressed mood most of the day, nearly every day
- Markedly diminshed interest or pleasure in all, or almost all, activities
- Decreased or increased appetite and weight
- Decreased (insomnia) or increased (hypersomnia) sleep

101

- Physical agitation (inability to sit still, hand wringing, pacing) or slowness (retardation) of activity
- Fatigue or loss of energy
- Feelings of worthlessness or excessive or inappropriate guilt
- Diminished ability to think or concentrate or unusual indecisiveness
- Recurrent thoughts of death or suicide

When a major depressive episode is accompanied by hallucinations or delusions, the major depressive disorder is a psychotic depression (**major depression with psychotic features**).

Another subtype of major depression is the **melancholic** type. This type of depression is very responsive to antidepressant medications and electroconvulsive therapy (ECT). In addition to the symptoms listed above, **major depression with melancholic features** is characterized by

- Depressed mood occurring more severely in the mornings
- Awaking early in the morning before the usual time and having difficulty going back to sleep
- Significant loss of appetite and weight loss
- A relatively fixed depressed mood that does not react to pleasurable events

Other Forms of Depression

Seasonal Affective Disorder (SAD)

For some people living in climates with marked seasonal changes of daylight, their mood may fluctuate with the seasons. Dark, dreary winter months may bring on annual depression that begins around October or November, with January and February generally being the worst months. The depression usually resolves with the coming of spring in March or April. This seasonal pattern of depression is called **seasonal affective disorder** (SAD) and has many of the symptoms of major depression, but the symptoms are usually not quite as severe.

Patients with mild seasonal affective disorder may respond simply to phototherapy, a treatment using ultraviolet lamps to simulate sunlight. In more severe seasonal depression, patients may need both phototherapy and antidepressant medications.

Dysthymia

Dysthymia is a milder form of depression that has an early onset, developing in childhood, adolescence, or early adulthood. The impairment is due to the continuous nature of the disorder rather than its severity in this form of mild, chronic depression. The depressed mood is often accompanied by feelings of inadequacy, poor self-esteem, self-deprecation, indecisiveness, poor concentration, pessimism regarding the future, a sense of hopelessness, overeating or poor appetite, hypersomnia or insomnia, and tiredness or lack of energy. Dysthymic patients often seen to be unhappy but may not be aware that they are depressed, for their symptoms are less intense than those of major depression. However, these patients are more prone to develop major depression.

TREATMENT

The primary medical treatments of depression are medications and ECT. Psychotherapy may be used in addition to medications or ECT to support treatment. With mild depression, some clinicians may elect to try psychotherapy first before prescribing medication.

Antidepressants

Antidepressants can be divided into two general groups: 1) the *earlier antidepressants*, which include the tricyclic and tetracyclic antidepressants (TCAs) and the monoamine oxidase inhibitors (MAOIs); and 2) the *newer antidepressants*, which include the selective serotonin reuptake inhibitors (SSRIs) and other antidepressants that do not fit into the categories above, such as bupropion (Wellbutrin SR), nefazodone (Serzone), and venlafaxine (Effexor XR).

Imipramine was one of the first antidepressants developed back in the late 1950s. Imipramine has a three-ring chemical structure, and hence it is known as a tricyclic antidepressant. Imipramine was followed by the development of other tricyclic antidepressants, including amitriptyline (Elavil) and desipramine (Norpramin). Today there are a total of nine tricyclic antidepressant and two tetracyclic (four-ring structure) antidepressants, which differ little from the tricyclic compounds in their mode of action and side effects. The tricyclic and tetracyclic antidepressants are effective antidepressants and were widely prescribed for many decades before they were superseded by a new generation of antidepressants, such as fluoxetine (Prozac). The newer antidepressants are not necessarily more effective than the TCAs, but they are safer and have fewer side effects than the older antidepressants.

Another class of antidepressants, developed around the same time as the TCAs, comprises the *monoamine oxidase inhibitors*. MAOI antidepressants include phenelzine (Nardil), tranylcypromine (Parnate), and isocarboxazid (Marplan). Selegiline (Eldepryl), a newer MAOI, was approved by the federal Food and Drug Administration for treatment of Parkinson's disease, but some psychiatrists prescribe it for treating depression as well. With the availability of new antidepressants, the use of MAOIs has been limited, because these agents present potentially dangerous interactions with other medications and certain foods.

With the introduction of fluoxetine, or Prozac, in the early 1990s, the treatment of depression was revolutionized by an antidepressant that was not only effective but highly tolerated by patients. Fluoxetine represented the first in its class that worked by selectively increasing the neurotransmitter of serotonin in the brain. Following fluoxetine, other similar antidepressants were synthesized, and collectively, they are known as *selective serotonin reuptake inhibitors*. These antidepressants *inhibit* the reuptake of released serotonin back into the nerve cells and thus boost neurotransmission of these neurons. Other SSRI antidepressants include citalopram (Celexa), escitalopram (Lexapro), fluvoxamine (Luvox), paroxetine (Paxil), and sertraline (Zoloft).

The other new antidepressants that are not neatly categorized into any one group include bupropion (Wellbutrin), nefazodone (Serzone), trazodone (Desyrel), venlafaxine (Effexor), and mirtazapine (Remeron). These agents are also called dual-action antidepressants because either they affect more than one neurotransmitter or they exert their action at different sites on nerve cells. For a discussion of the antidepressants, refer to *Part 3 (Information About Medications for Patients and Families)*.

Generally, patients are prescribed one of the SSRIs, especially if it is their first episode of major depression. The SSRIs are effective, well tolerated, easy to dose, and generally safe if overdose occurs. The SSRIs may be dosed once daily either in the morning or at bedtime. It usually takes about 2–4 weeks for the antidepressant to achieve full effects, and a therapeutic trial should last 4–8 weeks at the maximum dose. If the patient's depressive symptoms are still present after this period, switching to another SSRI may often produce improved response. If adequate response is not achieved after the second trial of an SSRI, the patient should be switched to an antidepressant in a different class (e.g., bupropion, venlafaxine, or a TCA) with a different mechanism of action.

If the third antidepressant trial fails and a patient's depression is deemed treatment-resistant, it then presents a treatment challenge for the physician. Some patients may benefit from lithium augmentation, in which lithium carbonate is added to boost the effect of the antidepressant. Some physicians may use a different augmentation strategy. Instead of lithium, liothyronine (T_3, Cytomel), a thyroid hormone, is added to the antidepressant, or another antidepressant from a different class is added to the first antidepressant (e.g., an SSRI and a TCA). Some physicians may use a mood stabilizer such as divalproex (Depakote) or carbamazepine (Tegretol) instead of lithium for augmentation. Patients whose depression continues to be refractory to treatment may benefit from treatment with an MAOI. For patients who are nonresponders to medications, ECT may be an option.

ECT

ECT can be a life-saving treatment for severe depression. It is often used for patients who have severe suicidal and/or delusional thoughts and for pregnant women who are severely depressed. When ECT achieves the desired response, it usually takes effect quicker than medications.

Psychotherapy

Supportive psychotherapy may be an invaluable adjunctive treatment for depression in addition to medication or ECT, but some patients with less severe depression (e.g., dysthymia) may respond to psychotherapy alone. The psychotherapist can help patients work through painful, internal conflicts of depression by examining the feelings of guilt, worthlessness, and hopelessness and eventually helping the patient regain confidence and self-esteem. One of the goals of psychotherapy is to identify the external and psychological stresses that may be causing the patient's distress and devise methods for coping with these issues. The clinician may help patients assess their problems with interpersonal relationships and help them recognize that these may be the result of their depressive illness rather than holding themselves responsible for their troubling consequences. This can enable them to deal with the embarrassment, fear, and anxiety of their depression. The clinician may also help patients recognize early signs of mood changes, so that early intervention may prevent a mild depression from becoming severe.

SUICIDE PREVENTION

When the patient is thinking or talking about suicide, seek help immediately.

- Call the physician or mental health worker, or go to a hospital emergency room to seek help.
- Call a suicide prevention center in your area.
- Talk to a friend, a relative, or a member of the clergy.
- In an emergency, if the individual is in the act of attempting suicide, call the police.

If you have any questions about this handout, please consult your physician.

SUPPORT AND ADVOCACY GROUPS

Depression Awareness, Recognition, and
   Treatment Program (D/ART)
National Institute of Mental Health
5600 Fishers Lane
Rockville, MD 20857
Phone: (800) 421-4211
Web site: http://www.nimh.nih.gov/
   HealthInformation/Depressionmenu.cfm

National Alliance for the Mentally Ill
Colonial Place Three
2107 Wilson Blvd., Suite 300
Arlington, VA 22201-3042
Phone: (800) 950-NAMI; (703) 524-7600
Web site: http://www.nami.org

National Foundation for Depressive Illness, Inc.
P.O. Box 2257
New York, NY 10116
Phone: (800) 239-1265
Web site: http://www.depression.org

Depressives Anonymous
329 E. 62nd Street, Suite 50
New York, NY 100021
Phone: (212) 689-2600

Depression After Delivery, Inc.
91 East Somerset Street
Raritan, NJ 08869
Phone: (800) 944-4PPD (4773) Information
Web site: www.depressionafterdelivery.com

INFORMATION ABOUT

OBSESSIVE-COMPULSIVE DISORDER

FOR PATIENTS AND FAMILIES

Obsessive-compulsive disorder (OCD) is a psychiatric illness with two essential features: obsessions and/or compulsions. **Obsessions** are recurrent, persistent, and intrusive thoughts, impulses, or images that cause marked anxiety, fear, and distress. The individual is aware that these obsessions are inappropriate and irrational and not simply due to excessive worries from situational problems. The obsessional thoughts, impulses, or images are recognized as originating internally and therefore provoke conflict and anxiety. However, the patient is powerless to control these obsessions. To deal with the internal conflicts, the individual tries to ignore, suppress, or neutralize the intrusive or inappropriate obsessions with other thoughts or actions.

Compulsions are repetitive, purposeful behaviors or mental acts (e.g., praying, counting, or repeating words silently) performed in response to decrease anxiety and distress associated with obsessions or to prevent obsessional thoughts. The individual uses repetitive, ritualistic behavior in attempt to neutralize the anxiety and distress provoked by the obsessions. Each ritual is repeated over and over again until there is some relief of the anxiety and distress. Unfortunately, the relief is temporary because as obsessive thoughts recur, compulsive behaviors are repeated.

DIAGNOSIS

The diagnosis of OCD is made on the basis of a person's having either obsessions *or* compulsions, or both, with symptoms that cause marked anxiety and distress, result in time-consuming rituals, or interfere with the person's normal activities, job, or relationships. During the course of illness, the person (except children) may recognize that the obsessions and compulsive behaviors are irrational, excessive, or inappropriate. However, the person is powerless to control them. The following obsessive and compulsive symptoms are commonly seen in patients with OCD:

- *Fear of contamination.* An excessive obsession or fear of contamination is often present, accompanied by hand washing or other cleaning activity. The symptoms are similar to those of phobias. There is anxiety and fear of dirt, germs, bodily waste or secretions, environmental contamination, animals, insects, and so on. Individuals are often concerned with becoming contaminated by touching objects or people. They may wear gloves to avoid germs or use tissue paper to pick up objects.
- *Washing and cleaning.* An indication of compulsive hand washing may be raw, chafed hands, sometimes to the point where the hands are cracked and bleeding. Individuals may bathe numerous times during the day. These rituals become more frequent and time-consuming as the disorder is exacerbated.
- *Irrational doubt and insecurity.* Individuals may possess obsessive thoughts that something terrible or harmful will happen. Consequently, compulsive activities are performed in response to relieve the anxiety and distress. Individuals are compelled to check constantly on their surroundings to feel secure. For example, before leaving the house, they may check all the locks on the doors and windows or other fixtures around the house, such as water faucets, appliances, and electrical switches. They may need to count the number of times that things must be checked, and only after a certain number of times will it be "all right." The time-consuming ritual often causes these individuals to be late for work, school, or appointments.
- *Need for symmetry and precision.* Individuals may have a need to arrange things and events in a precise order or place. Things must be made symmetrical, orderly, and precise. Tasks must be performed in a certain order and done precisely. When things are not in perfect order or alignment, there is discontent and tension.

- *Somatic.* Individuals may have excessive preoccupation with a part of their body, appearance, or developing illness or disease. This excessive somatic preoccupation is similar to that of patients with **hypochondriasis,** but what separates obsessive-compulsive patients is that they have other obsessions and compulsions.
- *Hoarding.* Individuals may collect things, generally of little value, and count and check that nothing is missing or has been thrown out.
- *Religious obsessions.* Individuals may obsess over their religious beliefs and moral values, devoting many hours of the day to ritualistic practices. They may see their suffering as a religious trial and their rituals as an obligation of their religious cause.

There are individuals who have **obsessive-compulsive personality disorder** (OCPD) and not OCD. Although the diagnostic names are similar, these two disorders are different from each other. Individuals with OCPD have a need for perfectionism and orderliness, but they are not out of control and do not experience as much as dysfunction related to obsessions and compulsive behavior as patients with OCD. They may be obstinate about perfectionism, orderliness, and cleanliness, but generally they do not show the compulsive behavior of OCD. In fact, OCPD rarely leads to OCD, bolstering the argument that these disorders are separate entities. Moreover, individuals with OCPD do not respond to medications.

COURSE OF ILLNESS

Typically, OCD begins during the late teens and early twenties, usually between the ages of 19 and 24. It affects males and females almost equally, although males tend to have the illness earlier. Generally, the onset of illness is gradual, but the disorder may develop suddenly, as well. Depression often coexists with OCD, and recurrent depression may be as high as 80% in patients with OCD.

CAUSE OR ETIOLOGY

OCD affects about 1%–2% of the general population. There is strong evidence from family studies that some aspects of the illness are hereditary. Studies have shown that up to 20% of immediate relatives of patients with OCD have obsessive-compulsive symptoms. There also appears to be a genetic relationship between individuals with OCD and Tourette's syndrome, a tic disorder. Children of a parent with Tourette's syndrome are more likely than the average person to develop OCD.

Advancements in the treatment of OCD provide the strongest evidence that the basis of the illness may be biochemical, and not merely behavioral. The biochemical model of OCD is focused on the brain neurotransmitter **serotonin.** Experts believe that OCD may be caused by disturbance in the level of serotonin or by disturbance in areas of the brain involving serotonin. Generally, antidepressants that increase the levels of serotonin in the brain are effective agents for treating OCD.

TREATMENT

Medications

Antidepressants that are effective for treating the symptoms of OCD are those that work by increasing levels of serotonin. These antidepressants include **clomipramine** (Anafranil), tricyclic antidepressants, and the **selective serotonin reuptake inhibitors** (SSRIs), which include **citalopram** (Celexa), **fluoxetine** (Prozac), **fluvoxamine** (Luvox), **escitalopram** (Lexapro), **paroxetine** (Paxil), and **sertraline** (Zoloft). Clomipramine, the first drug marketed for OCD, is associated with frequent side effects that limit its usefulness. The SSRIs are generally better tolerated by patients and are currently the preferred medications for treating OCD. Treating OCD with SSRI antidepressants generally requires higher doses than are used for depression and lengthy trials because the response is often delayed.

Psychotherapy

Behavior therapy, in conjunction with pharmacotherapy, has produced dramatic success in the treatment of OCD. Behavior therapy consists of *exposure* and *response prevention*. The technique of exposure and response prevention requires patients to identify and confront the situation or stimulus that evokes fear or anxiety and then teaches them how to prevent and refrain from the compulsive behavior. For example, the therapist may ask the patient to step on a crack, creating anxiety, and in turn help the individual to learn not to react to the situation. In time, the patient's anxiety dampens and the ritual of avoiding cracks decreases. The therapist may also teach the patient thought-stopping techniques to interrupt the obsessive thoughts once they are triggered.

In the beginning of behavior therapy, there may be periods of considerable fear and anxiety, as the patient attempts to confront the problem. However, patients who persevere with treatment generally have a remarkable rate of improvement.

If you have any questions about this handout, please consult your physician.

SUPPORT AND ADVOCACY GROUPS

Obsessive-Compulsive Foundation, Inc.
676 State Street
New Haven, CT 06511
Phone: (203) 401-2070
Web site: www.ocfoundation.org
Provides education to the public about OCD and related disorders and assistance to patients and family, and supports research into the causes and treatment of OCD and related disorders.

Anxiety Disorders Association of America
8730 Georgia Avenue, Suite 600
Silver Spring, MD 20910
Phone: (240) 485-1001
Web site: www.adaa.org
A nonprofit organization dedicated to promoting the education and awareness of anxiety disorder.

INFORMATION ABOUT

SCHIZOPHRENIA

FOR PATIENTS AND FAMILIES

Schizophrenia is a disease that produces a wide range of mental symptoms, but the hallmark of schizophrenia is **psychosis.** It is a psychotic disorder that is characterized by hallucinations, delusions, abnormal emotions, impaired thinking, and behavioral changes when the individual loses the ability to separate his or her thoughts and perceptions from reality of the external world. The symptoms of hallucinations, delusions, bizarre behavior, and thought disorder are also called **positive symptoms** of schizophrenia, because these symptoms are obviously abnormal or in excess of what is normal when emotions or behavior may be greatly exaggerated or inappropriate to the situation.

Delusions are false beliefs or perceptions about something or someone. For examples, a *grandiose delusion* is a belief by a person that he or she has extraordinary power or ability, and a *paranoid delusion* is a persecutory suspicion held by the person that someone or something is out to control or harm him or her.

Hallucinations are false sensations. They can be heard *(auditory)*, seen *(visual)*, smelled *(olfactory),* tasted *(gustatory),* or felt *(tactile).* Schizophrenic patients commonly have auditory hallucinations, particularly early in the course of illness. **Command hallucinations** command the individual to do something, which may be harmful to self or others.

A dimension of schizophrenia that is less obvious, but common, is the presence of impaired emotional responsiveness in schizophrenic patients. The deficit symptoms are called **negative symptoms** of schizophrenia. Negative symptoms are characterized by flat or blunted emotions, impoverishment of speech, loss of motivation and initiative, inability to experience or derive pleasure from daily life, and attention deficit. When patients experience negative symptoms, they show very little emotion and enthusiasm or derive little enjoyment or pleasure from life (**anhedonia**), and they have marked loss of energy to initiate any goal-directed behavior.

Psychosis is a clinical term to delineate a mixture of symptoms that must minimally include delusions and hallucinations. Besides schizophrenia, psychosis is associated with many other psychiatric disorders, including substance-induced psychosis, mania, and psychotic depression. However, schizophrenia is the most recognized of the psychotic disorders.

Other symptoms of schizophrenia include lack of insight and judgment, disorganized thinking, loss of interest in personal appearance and hygiene, and deterioration of social behavior. With poor insight, patients may not be compliant with taking medications because they do not think they are ill. Rates of alcohol and drug abuse are high among schizophrenic patients. Their susceptibility to substance abuse may stem from their lack of insight and judgment. Moreover, they may use alcohol and drugs to quiet their symptoms (e.g., voices) when they are not taking their medications. Disorganized thinking in patients with schizophrenia is distinct from their delusions and hallucinations, and schizophrenia is often characterized as a **thought disorder.** As a result, the content of their speech may be illogical, disorganized, loosely associated, and often bizarre. The deterioration of social behavior may result from the confluence of symptoms, and the patient becomes unkempt and odorous, ignores his or her social surroundings, and behaves inappropriately in public.

DIAGNOSIS AND SUBTYPES OF SCHIZOPHRENIA

Schizophrenia must fulfill several diagnostic criteria in the following categories: 1) characteristic symptoms, 2) duration, 3) social and occupational dysfunction, and 4) exclusion of other causes.

The diagnosis must have two or more of the following characteristic symptoms:

- Delusions
- Hallucinations
- Disorganized speech
- Grossly disorganized or catatonic behavior
- Negative symptoms

Symptoms must persist continuously for at least 6 months. Since the onset of symptoms, problems with interpersonal relationships, at work, or at school have significantly disrupted the patient's life. The patient's disturbance is not due to other causes, such as substance-induced psychosis, a medical condition, or another psychiatric disorder.

Five subtypes of schizophrenia are recognized:

- *Catatonic* schizophrenia is associated with disturbance of movement. Movement may be decreased to the point that the individual is unable to speak (mutism), assumes strange postures, or becomes rigid. Or, the movements may be excessive, purposeless activity and totally dissociated from the individual's surroundings.
- *Paranoid* schizophrenia is defined by the predominance of one or more delusions or auditory hallucinations, which are usually persecutory in nature. The paranoid delusions and hallucinations are usually organized and systemized (there is a theme to them) and relatively consistent. Individuals with paranoid schizophrenia are often angry, argumentative, and violent.
- *Disorganized* schizophrenia is characterized by disorganized speech and behavior. The delusions and hallucinations are fragmented and disorganized and do not have the coherent theme found in paranoid schizophrenia. Hence the content of the speech of patients with the disorganized type is extremely loose and difficult to follow. Their behavior seems purposeless, silly, and childlike.
- *Undifferentiated* schizophrenia is a subtype for those symptoms that do not fit into the other categories.
- *Residual* schizophrenia is a category that describes the situation in which a patient's psychotic symptoms (i.e., positive symptoms) have subsided but residual symptoms (i.e., negative symptoms), such as emotional blunting, social withdrawal, illogical thinking, disturbance in thinking, or eccentric behavior, persist.

However, subtyping is not always accurate or reliable, because a patient's symptoms may change over the course of illness and, in many cases, fit several subtypes. It is practical to describe the patient's prominent symptoms.

COURSE OF ILLNESS

Schizophrenia is one of the most devastating mental illnesses that can afflict a person, leading to a lifetime of debilitations. In the United States, schizophrenia affects about 1%–1.5% of the population. Approximately 3 to 5 million people may have schizophrenia at any given time. It affects men and women equally, but men tend to have an earlier onset than women. The onset for men is usually between the ages of 15 and 25; for women, in contrast, the onset is usually between the ages of 25 and 35.

Usually, the onset of schizophrenia is gradual, with a premonitory, or *prodromal*, phase before there is evidence of psychosis. The patient may withdraw from friends and family, become less communicative, display peculiar changes in behavior, have blunted emotions, and express strange ideas or become excessively religious. By themselves, none of these early symptoms fulfills the diagnostic criteria for schizophrenia. When psychotic symptoms initially appear, it is apparent that the individual is psychotic, and a clinical diagnosis of schizophrenia can be made. The psychotic phase of the disease is also called the *active phase* of schizophrenia. During a psychotic break, or episode, the individual may have a wide range of positive symptoms, including hallucinations and delusions. As positive symptoms subside with medical intervention, the individual enters into the *residual phase* of the illness. During the residual phase, psychotic symptoms may be present, but at a lower intensity than during the active phase, with negative symptoms being most prominent.

The clinical course and outcome in schizophrenia vary with patients. Some patients may go into remission and are relatively free of symptoms, while others may continue to have some residual symptoms. Furthermore, those who have severe, unremitting psychosis may require hospitalization in mental institutions.

Unfortunately, schizophrenia is a chronic illness, and for most patients the illness may wax and wane for many years. Some patients may remain in remission and symptom-free for years. For the vast majority of patients, however, the cycle of relapse and remission is the general course of schizophrenia. Over time, the morbidity of the disease increases as patients' residual symptoms become more persistent and their level of functioning further decreases.

The risk of suicide is high, particularly early in the course of schizophrenia. About one-third of patients will attempt suicide, and about 1% will take their lives. However, the risk of suicide apparently decreases over time as the individual adapts to the illness.

CAUSE OR ETIOLOGY

The causes of schizophrenia are unknown, but there is strong evidence that some aspects of the illness are hereditary, or genetically linked. The consensus among experts is that schizophrenia is inherited and that an individual carries a genetic predisposition for the disease. However, the disease is not manifested unless other factors come into play to trigger the expression of the genes that code for the disease. These factors may be biological or may be related to the individual's psychosocial environment. For example, family members or friends can often identify some event or stressor in the patient's past that led to the "nervous breakdown," which was subsequently diagnosed as schizophrenia. And according to the experts, the individual with a heavy genetic load (genes) for the disease has greater susceptibility and vulnerability for developing schizophrenia at a younger age.

The pattern of inheritance in schizophrenia comes from family studies. Siblings of schizophrenic patients have a 10% chance of developing schizophrenia. If one of the siblings with schizophrenia is an identical twin, the other has a 46% chance of developing the illness, whereas in fraternal twins the rate is only 14%. In families in which one parent is afflicted with schizophrenia, there is a 5%–6% chance the children may develop the disease. However, when both parents have schizophrenia, the risk of their children developing the disease increases to 46%. The exact role that heredity plays in schizophrenia is unknown because the disease is confounded by many factors, including those exerted by the individual's environment.

TREATMENT

Medication

The standard treatment for schizophrenia is antipsychotic medications. **Chlorpromazine** (Thorazine), the first antipsychotic introduced to psychiatry over 50 years ago, changed the course of treating schizophrenia and mental illness in general. The next major breakthrough came almost 20 years later with the discovery of **clozapine** (Clozaril), the first in the class of a second generation of novel antipsychotics. In the past 10 years, five other second-generation antipsychotics have been introduced: **risperidone** (Risperdal), **olanzapine** (Zyprexa), **quetiapine** (Seroquel), **ziprasidone** (Geodon), and **aripiprazole** (Abilify). These antipsychotics represent a major advancement in the treatment of schizophrenia, and they are the mainstay of treatment for schizophrenia, replacing the first-generation antipsychotics such as chlorpromazine, **haloperidol** (Haldol), and **fluphenazine** (Prolixin). For a discussion of antipsychotic medications, see *Part 3 (Information About Medications for Patients and Families)*.

When clozapine was introduced for treatment of schizophrenia, it proved to be a remarkable drug. Clinical studies showed that about one-third of the patients who did not respond (treatment-resistant) to other antipsychotics improved when they were treated with clozapine. Clozapine, however, is reserved as a second-line treatment when patients do not respond to two or more trials of other antipsychotics. Clozapine is not widely used because it is associated with a rare, but potentially fatal, reaction that destroys an individual's white blood cells (**agranulocytosis**). Clozapine requires weekly or biweekly blood testing to monitor the patient's white blood cells. The medication is interrupted or discontinued when the number of white blood cells drops. Many patients find it difficulty to follow a regimen of weekly or biweekly monitoring. However, for patients who benefit from clozapine, the successful outcome may convince them that the inconvenience of routine blood tests is worth the effort.

The other second-generation antipsychotics differ little in their ability to treat schizophrenia, and for the most part, their differences lie in their side effects. Unlike clozapine, aripiprazole, olanzapine, risperidone, quetiapine, and ziprasidone have not been associated with agranulocytosis. Therefore, they do not require routine laboratory monitoring of white blood cells. These agents have become first-line therapies for treating schizophrenia; the first-generation antipsychotics are relegated to backup therapies. A physician's decision to use one antipsychotic over another may be based on the patient's previous response to medications or on the side-effect profile of the antipsychotic that is most compatible for the patient.

Haloperidol, fluphenazine, and risperidone are also available in long-acting injections for intramuscular administration. Haloperidol and fluphenazine come in **decanoate** injections—**haloperidol decanoate** (Haldol Decanoate) and **fluphenazine decanoate** (Prolixin Decanoate)—whereas risperidone injection (**Risperdal Consta**), using modern technology, incorporates the drug into microspheres. The injected antipsychotic is slowly absorbed from the muscle tissues. This gives haloperidol decanoate a duration of action of about 4 weeks, and fluphenazine decanoate and Risperdal Consta a duration of action of about 2 weeks. The long-acting injections provide an alternative to taking oral medications and are particularly helpful for patients who have difficulty adhering to a medication schedule.

Unlike the older antipsychotics, the second-generation agents have a much lower propensity to cause neurologic side effects that result in intolerable movement disorders. Because of the neurological side effects they produce, the typical antipsychotics are also known as **neuroleptics**. With few side effects, patients are usually more compliant with taking atypical antipsychotics.

In an acutely psychotic state, patients are managed in an acute inpatient psychiatric hospital where they can be closely monitored. During an acute episode, higher doses of antipsychotic medications may be needed. Moreover, antipsychotic medications in liquid and injectable forms may be administered to patients who are too agitated or noncompliant with taking medications. Once psychotic symptoms are under control and the patient is ready to be discharged, the physician will usually have the patient continue taking the antipsychotic medication. The patient begins taking a maintenance dose of the antipsychotic, which may be lower than the previous inpatient dose. Often, patients (and family members) ask how long they must continue taking the antipsychotic medications. Generally, patients benefit from continuing treatment to prevent relapse. If it is the patient's first psychotic episode, maintenance treatment for at least 1–2 years is recommended to prevent emergence of symptoms. On the other hand, if the patient has had multiple episodes, the patient may need life-long antipsychotic therapy, because the risk of relapse is higher.

Psychosocial Support

Although antipsychotic medications are the foundation for treating schizophrenia, providing the patient with psychosocial support is also important for improving outcome and preventing relapse. Psychosocial support is directed toward helping the patient and family members in the following areas:

- Learning and understanding schizophrenia and coming to terms with it
- Learning to recognize, avoid, and cope with stressful situations in preventing relapse
- Teaching the patient living and social skills, depending on the level of function
- Providing medication education to help the patient (and family members) understand his or her medications, the side effects of the medications, and the importance of medication compliance
- Providing social services to the patient and family members to ensure the patient receives adequate mental health care and community services
- Preventing the patient from seeking high-risk behavior, such as using drugs and alcohol

If you have any questions about this handout, please consult your physician.

SUPPORT AND ADVOCACY GROUPS

National Alliance for the Mental Ill (NAMI)
Colonial Place Three
2107 Wilson Blvd., Suite 300
Arlington, VA 22201-3042
Phone: (800) 950-NAMI (6264); (703) 524-7600
Web site: www.nami.org
Provides self-help and advocacy for persons with mental illness and their families.

National Mental Health Consumers' Self-Help
Clearinghouse
1211 Chestnut Street, Suite 1207
Philadelphia, PA 19107
Phone: (800) 553-4KEY (4539); (215) 751-1810
Web site: www.mhselfhelp.org
Connects individuals to self-help and advocacy resources.

National Alliance for Research on Schizophrenia
and Depression
60 Cutter Mill Road, Suite 404
Great Neck, NY 11021
Phone: (800) 829-8289
Web site: www.narsad.org
A donor-supported organization whose mission is to raise funds for scientific research on psychiatric brain disorders.

INFORMATION ABOUT

TARDIVE DYSKINESIA

FOR PATIENTS AND FAMILIES

Tardive dyskinesia (TD) is a disorder of abnormal involuntary movements produced by long-term use of antipsychotic (also called **neuroleptic**) medications. As the term *tardive* implies, the resultant disorder is a delayed adverse reaction from prolonged exposure to antipsychotic medications. The abnormal movements (dyskinesia) are involuntary and irregular. They usually involve the mouth, tongue, and, less commonly, arms and legs. Often TD involves more than one area of the body. The most commonly observed movement abnormalities are seen with the tongue (darting, writhing, and twisting movements and repeated protrusions) and fingers and hands ("pill-rolling" and hand clenching). Movements of the mouth include chewing, lip puckering, and lateral jaw movements. As the dyskinesia becomes more severe, the patient may have twisting of the trunk, thrusting of the pelvis, respiratory grunting, and arm and leg movements. When the movements are rapid, jerky, nonrepetitive, and seemingly purposeful, they are called **choreiform**. When the movements are rhythmic, continuous, slow, sinuous, and without purpose, they are called **athetoid**. A combination of choreiform and athetoid movements is called **choreoathetoid** movements.

Long-term use of antipsychotic medications may also cause a chronic disorder of muscle tone, called **tardive dystonia**. The involuntary slow contraction and twisting of particular muscle groups produce dystonic movements and abnormal postures. The condition may range from mild to severe, and in more severe cases, tardive dystonia may be painful, bizarre, and debilitating.

The severity of TD may range from mild to moderate tongue and finger movements to severe, disfiguring, and incapacitating movements of the extremities. In mild cases of TD, the visible movements are merely seen as peculiar tics and restlessness, but in severe cases the severity of abnormal movements may cause social or functional problems.

RISK OF TARDIVE DYSKINESIA

The risk of TD can be estimated statistically from studies with patients exposed to antipsychotic medications, but it is impossible to predict which patients will develop dyskinesia from antipsychotics. However, there are certain risk factors associated with developing TD from exposure to antipsychotic medications.

- *Length of treatment.* The longer a patient is treated with antipsychotic medications, the greater the risk of developing TD. The best available data suggest that for the first 5 years of treatment, on average, there is about 4%–5% per year cumulative risk of developing TD. Some patients may develop TD within less than 1 year of exposure to antipsychotics, but for the majority of patients the risk is correlated with duration of antipsychotic treatment over many years.
- *Age and sex.* The risk of TD increases with age—in terms of not only incidence but also severity and persistence of abnormal movements. The age of the patient is perhaps the single most important risk factor. In elderly patients who have not been previously treated with antipsychotics, TD generally develops more rapidly and at lower doses than in younger patients. Moreover, women appear to be at greater risk than men of similar age and cumulative drug exposure, and they are also more likely to develop more severe forms of dyskinesia.
- *Type of antipsychotic medication.* The older, first-generation antipsychotics are associated with a higher incidence of TD than the newer, second-generation antipsychotic medications. From clinical studies, it is well established that the first-generation antipsychotics, such as **chlorpromazine** (Thorazine), **haloperidol** (Haldol), **fluphenazine** (Prolixin), and others, induce TD. However, it is not clear if one anti-

113

psychotic is more likely than another to produce TD. The second-generation antipsychotics, however, may have a lower incidence of TD. In over 30 years of experience with **clozapine** (Clozaril), the first of the second-generation antipsychotics, it rarely caused TD. The risks of developing TD from other second-generation antipsychotic medications—**aripiprazole** (Abilify), **olanzapine** (Zyprexa), **quetiapine** (Seroquel) **risperidone** (Risperdal), and **ziprasidone** (Geodon), all relatively new antipsychotic medications—are not presently known. However, these agents are expected to have a similarly low risk for TD.

- *Other associated risk factors.* Patients with a mood disorder (e.g., bipolar disorder or major depression) appear to be at greater risk for developing TD when treated with antipsychotic medications.

TREATMENT ISSUES

Because TD is caused by chronic use of antipsychotic medications, cessation of these medications, if possible, is the best course of treatment. In fact, up to one-third of patients who develop TD may become symptom-free within 3 months of discontinuing antipsychotic medications, and up to 60% of patients who discontinue antipsychotic medications for 5 years may see their symptoms go into remission.

Unfortunately, for most patients discontinuation of their antipsychotic medication is not a viable option, since most patients will relapse shortly without treatment. Various medications have been use to treat TD with equivocal success. **Antiparkinson medications** (e.g., Cogentin), used to treat Parkinson's disease and movement disorders induced by antipsychotic medications, are not effective for treating TD. In fact, these medications often make TD worse. **Clonidine** (Catapres) and **propranolol** (Inderal)—commonly used antihypertensive medications and widely used in other areas of medicine—may attenuate the abnormal movements for some patients but are generally not successful for treating most cases of TD. High doses of **vitamin E** (up to 1,600 IU/day) may help control the abnormal movements to some extent, but its benefit is inconclusive. Patients with TD should be offered a trial, since the use of vitamin E is relatively benign.

Many physicians may use clozapine to suppress the abnormal movements of TD. In fact, clozapine may have some benefit in treating TD. In several studies, when patients with TD were switched to clozapine, some had remarkable improvements of their abnormal movements.

Currently, physicians generally use the second-generation antipsychotics as first-line treatment for psychotic disorders. As these newer medications replace the older antipsychotics, we may see the incidence of TD decline dramatically in the future.

If you have any questions about this handout, please consult your physician.

SUPPORT AND ADVOCACY GROUPS

National Alliance for Research on
  Schizophrenia and Depression
60 Cutter Mill Road, Suite 404
Great Neck, NY 11021
Phone: (800) 829-8289
Web site: www.narsad.org
A donor-supported organization whose mission is to raise funds for scientific research on psychiatric brain disorders.

Tardive Dyskinesia / Tardive Dystonia
  National Association
4424 University Way, N.E.
Seattle, WA 98145-0732
Phone: (206) 522-3166
Seeks to promote education and understanding of tardive dyskinesia and tardive dystonia.

Part 3: Information About Medications for Patients and Families

INFORMATION ABOUT

ARIPIPRAZOLE (ABILIFY)

FOR PATIENTS AND FAMILIES

Aripiprazole (Abilify) is an antipsychotic medication used in the treatment of psychotic disorders, including schizophrenia, schizoaffective disorder, psychotic depression, and acute mania in bipolar disorder. Aripiprazole is a second-generation antipsychotic, a new class of medicines with actions different from those of older, first-generation antipsychotics such as **chlorpromazine** (Thorazine) and **haloperidol** (Haldol). The newer second-generation antipsychotics are more effective than the first-generation antipsychotics in reducing "negative" symptoms of schizophrenia. Negative symptoms are characterized by apathy, lack of motivation, flat emotional expression, depression, and withdrawal and isolation from people. Furthermore, the second-generation antipsychotics at standard doses rarely induce side effects associated with movement disorders, such as extrapyramidal symptoms (EPS) and tardive dyskinesia (TD). This is a very important distinction between the new and older antipsychotics.

Aripiprazole is marketed as the brand **Abilify.** It is available in 10-, 15-, 20-, and 30-mg tablets.

HOW ARIPIPRAZOLE IS PRESCRIBED

The recommended starting dose is 10–15 mg administered in a once-a-day schedule, preferably at bedtime. The dosage may be increased up to a maximum of 30 mg/day. Dosage increases should not be made sooner than 2 weeks to allow the medication to achieve optimal effects.

PROPER USE OF YOUR MEDICATION

Storing Your Medication

- Keep your medication in a tamper-resistant vial and out of reach of children.
- Store your medication so that it is kept from excessive heat, moisture, and direct light.
- Keep your medication in its original prescription vial with the label intact to prevent others from taking the medication inadvertently.

Taking Your Medication

- Take your medication as instructed by your physician. Do not abruptly stop taking your medication without telling your physician. Discontinuation of your medication may result in relapse.
- If you miss a dose, take it as soon as possible. However, if it is near the time of your next dose, skip the dose you missed and go back to your regular dosing schedule, but do not double-up the dose.
- Aripiprazole may be taken with food or without food. If it upsets your stomach, it may be best to take it with food.

Use of Alcohol and Other Medications

Individuals should refrain from using alcohol while taking aripiprazole. When alcohol is combined with aripiprazole, sedation and drowsiness, common side effects of the medication, may be made significantly worse. This may impair judgment, thinking, and coordination and, therefore, the ability to perform tasks. Some medications, including over-the-counter medicines, may interact with aripiprazole. The drug interaction may *lower* the blood level of the affected drug and decrease the drug's effectiveness; or, it may *elevate* the blood level of the affected drug and cause toxicity. When certain drugs are combined with aripiprazole, they may make some side effects worse. Inform your doctor of all the prescription and over-the-counter medications you are taking. If you have any questions or concerns about your medications, consult your physician or pharmacist.

POSSIBLE SIDE EFFECTS

- *Sedation and drowsiness.* Sedation and drowsiness are the most common complaints expressed by patients taking aripiprazole, especially immediately after starting therapy. These side effects eventually subside as the patient develops tolerance to the medication.

- *Orthostatic hypotension.* Aripiprazole may oppose the body's ability to elevate blood pressure in response to a change in position. If the blood pressure cannot increase in time to compensate for the change in position as the individual rises from a lying or sitting position, **orthostatic hypotension** ensues. As a result, the individual feels light-headed and dizzy, has a rapid heart rate, and may faint and fall. To prevent orthostatic hypotension after sitting for long periods or when rising out of bed, the patient should rise slowly to allow blood pressure to adjust gradually. Orthostatic hypotension from aripiprazole is usually mild, and patients generally adapt to it after the first or second week of therapy. Some medications, such as those used to lower blood pressure, may make orthostatic hypotension worse when combined with aripiprazole. If the problem is severe, the physician may lower the dose or change to another medication to correct it.

- *Gastrointestinal side effects.* Nausea, vomiting, constipation, and loss of appetite are some of the gastrointestinal side effects experienced by patients taking aripiprazole, especially at the onset of therapy. These side effects are usually mild and become less bothersome as the patient develops tolerance to them.

- *Weight gain.* Aripiprazole induces very little weight gain compared with other antipsychotics such as clozapine and olanzapine. However, some patients may experience weight gain when taking aripiprazole. Patients should consult their physician if excessive weight gain becomes problematic.

- *Extrapyramidal side effects.* Antipsychotic-induced neurologic side effects that cause movement disorders are commonly known as **extrapyramidal symptoms**. EPS include akathisia, Parkinson-like symptoms, and dystonia. Conventional antipsychotic medications such as haloperidol frequently induce EPS. Aripiprazole, on the other hand, *rarely* causes EPS, and when EPS do occur, it is usually at higher doses. In clinical trials, the incidence of reported EPS for aripiprazole-treated patients was similar to that for placebo.

     Some patients may experience **akathisia** from aripiprazole, which is described as an inner feeling of restlessness, expressed by constant pacing, inability to sit still, nervousness, and even agitation. Reducing the dose of antipsychotic is usually the most effective treatment for akathisia. If reducing the dose is not an option, the physician may add another medication to treat akathisia. The agent commonly prescribed is **propranolol** (Inderal), which belongs to a class of medicines called **beta-blockers.** Beta-blocking agents have many different uses, but they are primarily prescribed for treating heart disease and hypertension.

     Patients taking higher doses of aripiprazole may develop **Parkinson-like symptoms,** which are similar to the symptoms of **Parkinson's disease.** Patients with Parkinson-like symptoms may have a tremor of the fingers and hands, muscle stiffness, a shuffle when walking, stooped posture, drooling, and a mask-like face. These side effects are reversible and effectively treated with anticholinergic agents such as **benztropine** (Cogentin), **diphenhydramine** (Benadryl), or **trihexyphenidyl** (Artane).

Dystonia is another type of movement disorder induced by antipsychotics, although it rarely occurs with aripiprazole. As with all antipsychotics, there is the potential for dystonia. This reaction is manifested as a sudden spasm of the muscles of the tongue, jaw, or neck. It is not an allergic reaction, but it can be very frightening for the patient. The patient should seek immediate medical attention, because a dystonic reaction can be reversed rapidly with an intramuscular injection of benztropine or diphenhydramine.

- *Other possible side effects.* Headaches, stuffy noses, skin rash, and flulike symptoms are other possible side effects of aripiprazole.

Warning: Aripiprazole may cause drowsiness and sedation and impair physical coordination and mental alertness. Until you are sure that these side effects will not impair your ability to perform daily tasks, it is important to avoid potentially dangerous activities, such as driving a car or operating machinery.

POSSIBLE ADVERSE REACTIONS

- *Tardive dyskinesia (TD).* TD is by definition a late-onset abnormal, involuntary movement disorder. It is potentially an irreversible condition with symptoms that commonly include "pill-rolling" movements of the fingers, darting and writhing movements of the tongue, lip puckering, facial grimacing, and other irregular movements. It is suggested that the risk for developing TD with conventional antipsychotics is associated with the duration and amount of antipsychotic the patient was exposed to over the life of treatment. As the duration and amount of exposure to antipsychotics increase, so does the patient's risk of developing TD.

  The incidence of TD from atypical antipsychotics, however, is much lower than that from conventional antipsychotics. Because aripiprazole was recently introduced to the U.S. market, experience to date with the drug is limited. However, it is expected that the risk of developing TD from aripiprazole is very low. As with all antipsychotics, though, routine monitoring for TD is important.

- *Seizures.* Aripiprazole may lower the seizure threshold and precipitate seizures in susceptible individuals, particularly those with a history of seizure disorders. However, the risk of seizures is very low. Aripiprazole should be used cautiously in patients with a history of seizures.

- *Neuroleptic malignant syndrome (NMS).* NMS is a rare, toxic reaction to antipsychotics, including aripiprazole. The symptoms are severe muscle stiffness, rigidity, elevated body temperature, increased heart rate and blood pressure, irregular pulse, and sweating. NMS can lead to delirium and coma. It may be fatal if medical intervention is not immediately provided. There are no tests that can predict if an individual may be susceptible to developing NMS when exposed to an antipsychotic. Hence, NMS must be recognized early because it is a medical emergency that requires immediate discontinuation of the antipsychotic, hospitalization, and intensive medical treatment.

- *Heatstroke.* Antipsychotics, including aripiprazole, may induce heatstroke, resulting in elevation of high body temperature and dehydration. High body temperature is potentially dangerous if the temperature is not lowered. It usually occurs in patients who are exposed to very warm temperatures and who become dehydrated. To prevent heatstroke, patients should drink plenty of fluids and stay in air-conditioned environments during hot weather.

USE IN PREGNANCY AND BREAST FEEDING

Aripiprazole is classified in **Category C** of the U.S. Food and Drug Administration (FDA) Pregnancy Risk Categories. There are no studies, nor is there information, on the extent of risk of aripiprazole during pregnancy.

The risk to the fetus is unknown. In animal studies, however, some fetal abnormalities were found after maternal exposure to aripiprazole. Interpretation of these animal studies in regard to human risk is unclear. Women who are pregnant, or who plan to become pregnant, should not take aripiprazole. However, if the risk of not treating poses a greater danger for the mother and child, the benefits of treatment with aripiprazole may outweigh any unknown risks.

It is not known whether aripiprazole is excreted into human breast milk. It is recommended that women taking aripiprazole not breastfeed. If the drug is excreted in breast milk, it may have harmful effects on the infant when ingested.

If you have any questions about this handout, please consult your physician.

INFORMATION ABOUT

CLOZAPINE (CLOZARIL)

FOR PATIENTS AND FAMILIES

Clozapine (Clozaril) was used in Europe for many decades before it become available in the United States in 1989. Clozapine is one of the earlier second-generation antipsychotics that represent a new class of medicines with actions uniquely different from those of the older, first-generation antipsychotics. Clozapine and other second-generation antipsychotics have given patients greater hope and treatment options for such devastating illnesses as schizophrenia and bipolar disorder. The second-generation antipsychotics are more effective than the earlier antipsychotics, such as haloperidol, in reducing "negative" symptoms of schizophrenia. Negative symptoms are characterized by inappropriate expression of emotions, such as apathy, lack of motivation, flat emotional expression, restriction in thought and speech, and isolation and withdrawal from people. Moreover, the neurologic side effects that result in movement disorders are extremely rare with clozapine.

Patients who have had poor response to other antipsychotics may benefit from clozapine. In numerous cases, patients who were treatment-resistant to antipsychotics had a dramatic response to clozapine. Also, patients who have developed intractable movement disorders from antipsychotics, such as tardive dyskinesia (TD), may benefit from clozapine because it rarely causes these side effects.

Clozapine is marketed in the United States as the brand Clozaril, but the drug is also available from other generic manufacturers. Clozapine is available only in tablet form, in 25- and 100-mg strengths.

HOW CLOZAPINE IS PRESCRIBED

Clozapine is not a medication that is easy to prescribe, despite its tremendous benefits. Clozapine may induce a serious drug reaction (see "Possible Adverse Reactions"—**agranulocytosis**), so patients must be monitored closely. Before clozapine may be dispensed, the pharmacist must enroll the patient into one of three clozapine national registries, depending on which manufacturer is used. The registry monitors and tracks the patient during the course of clozapine treatment.

Before clozapine is initiated, pretreatment laboratory tests are needed, if they were not previously done. Blood tests include a complete blood cell count (CBC), which tests for white blood cells (WBCs), as well as granulocytes, and a chemistry panel. Granulocytes, a type of WBC, play a vital role in the body's defense against infections.

The usual starting dose for clozapine is 25 mg once or twice a day. The dose is increased by 25–50 mg once a day every 3–4 days until the desired clinical response is achieved. The dosage varies from patient to patient and may range from 300 to 600 mg/day. However, some patients may require dosages higher than 600 mg/day, sometimes up to a maximum of 900 mg/day.

The required protocol for clozapine monitoring involves a weekly blood test to monitor the patient's WBCs and granulocytes. The results of the tests are sent to the physician and pharmacist, who are responsible for reviewing them. When the test results are normal, the pharmacist is allowed to dispense a 1-week supply of clozapine. The following week, the procedure is repeated. The pharmacist is also responsible for sending the results of the blood count to the patient's registry. If weekly WBC counts are normal after the first 6 months of clozapine, the patient then requires monitoring only every other week and can receive a 2-week supply of medication thereafter.

PROPER USE OF YOUR MEDICATION

Storing Your Medication

- Keep your medication in a tamper-resistant vial and out of reach of children.
- Store your medication so that it is kept from excessive heat, moisture, and direct light.
- Keep your medication in its original prescription vial with the label intact to prevent others from taking the medication inadvertently.
- Do not use the medication past the expiration date on the prescription label.

Taking Your Medication

- It is important that you take clozapine according to your doctor's instructions. Do not abruptly stop taking your clozapine. Abrupt discontinuation of your medication may result in relapse. Clozapine should be decreased gradually before discontinuation.
- If you miss a dose, take it as soon as possible. However, if it is 1–2 hours before your next dose, skip the dose you missed and go back to your regular dosing schedule, but do not double-up the dose.
- It is very important that you obtain your weekly or biweekly blood test. Keep in mind that your clozapine can only be dispensed when you get your blood test.

Use of Alcohol and Other Medications

Individuals should refrain from alcohol consumption while taking clozapine. When the two are combined, sedation may increase significantly. Before consuming alcohol, consult your physician.

Some medications, including over-the-counter medicines, may interact with clozapine and make the side effects worse. Inform your doctor of all the prescription and over-the-counter medications that you are taking. If you have any questions or concerns about your medications, consult your physician or pharmacist.

POSSIBLE SIDE EFFECTS

- *Drowsiness and sedation.* Clozapine often produces significant sedation and drowsiness at the start of therapy, but these effects will usually subside when the patient develops tolerance to the medication. Taking a larger portion of a divided dose at bedtime may mitigate daytime drowsiness.
- *Hypersalivation.* Clozapine may increase saliva production. Although some patients have a dry mouth when taking clozapine, others find that the clozapine increases salivation, especially during sleep. Hypersalivation may decrease during the course of therapy. If the problem persists, an *anticholinergic* agent, such as **benztropine** (Cogentin) or **diphenhydramine** (Benadryl), may decrease saliva production.
- *Orthostatic hypotension.* Low blood pressure due to a postural change is known as **orthostatic hypotension**. Clozapine may oppose the body's ability to elevate blood pressure in response to a change in position. If the blood pressure cannot elevate in time to compensate for the change in position as the individual rises from a lying or sitting position, orthostatic hypotension ensues. As a result, the individual feels light-headed and dizzy, has a rapid heart rate, and may faint and fall. By learning to get up slowly to allow the blood pressure to adjust, the patient can avoid or minimize orthostatic hypotension. This practice is particularly important when getting up after sitting for long periods or when rising from bed. Usually the individual adapts to orthostatic hypotension. If the problem is severe, lowering the dose or switching to another medication may be necessary.

- *Dry mouth.* Although some patients may experience excessive saliva production, clozapine may also produce a dry mouth. Often this side effect subsides when the dose of clozapine has been stabilized and the patient develops tolerance to the medication. Chewing sugarless gum or sucking on sugarless candy may provide some relief for the patient.
- *Constipation.* Clozapine may slow gastrointestinal movement and cause constipation. To prevent constipation, the patient should increase fluid intake, eat a high-fiber diet, and exercise regularly. A bulk laxative, such as Metamucil, or a stool softener, such as docusate, is helpful when needed for constipation.
- *Blurred vision.* Clozapine may cause blurred vision and impair accommodation (ability of the eye to adjust when looking at close objects). If this occurs, the patient should inform his or her physician. Lowering the dose will usually eliminate this problem.
- *Urinary retention.* This side effect may be due to clozapine's effects on the bladder, decreasing urine flow or causing difficulty in urinating. Men with enlarged prostate glands may be more sensitive to this side effect. When urinary retention occurs, the patient should inform his or her physician. Lowering the dose may reverse this side effect.
- *Weight gain.* Weight gain is a common side effect of clozapine, and some patients experience significant weight gain from the medication. The major concerns from excessive weight are the health consequences to the patient, including the potential for developing diabetes and cardiovascular disease. Furthermore, patients may stop taking their medication when they become self-conscious about their weight. If the weight gain becomes problematic, the patient should consult with his or her physician. Both physician and patient can mutually agree on a supervised program, including diet and exercise, to reduce and control weight.
- *Altered glucose metabolism and diabetes.* Atypical antipsychotics may affect the way the body handles glucose, perhaps by decreasing the body's sensitivity to insulin. As a result, glucose levels in the blood may be elevated (**hyperglycemia**). Cases of drug-induced **diabetes** have been reported with two atypical antipsychotics: clozapine and olanzapine.
- *Photosensitivity.* Clozapine may increase photosensitivity. That is, clozapine may increase a person's sensitivity to sunlight and susceptibility to sunburn. Preventative measures include using sunscreen and avoiding excessive exposure to sunlight.
- *Extrapyramidal side effects.* Movement disorders caused by antipsychotics, resulting from their neurologic side effects, are commonly called **extrapyramidal symptoms** (EPS). Typical antipsychotic medications frequently induce EPS, whereas atypical antipsychotics infrequently produce these side effects. Clozapine, an atypical antipsychotic, rarely induces EPS, if at all, and this is a distinct advantage of clozapine over the conventional antipsychotics.

POSSIBLE ADVERSE REACTIONS

- *Agranulocytosis.* This is a condition in which the body's WBCs and granulocytes are significantly diminished in circulation. Granuloctyes, a type of WBC, play an important role in the body's defense in fighting and preventing infections. When granulocytes are dramatically diminished (**agranulocytosis**), a person becomes susceptible to life-threatening infections because the body's immunity is compromised.

    Patients taking clozapine have an estimated risk of 1% (1 in 100 patients) of developing agranulocytosis. This risk appears to be the greatest during the first 6 months of therapy. When agranulotcytosis is detected early, and with timely discontinuation of clozapine, the patient should recover completely without serious consequences. Unfortunately, there have been deaths from clozapine-induced agranulocytosis. Because of this potentially fatal adverse reaction, patients are required under the clozapine monitoring system to have their WBC and granulocyte counts checked at least once a week. The requirement has been relaxed to WBC and granulocyte counts every 2 weeks if blood test results are normal after the first 6 months of therapy.

- *Tardive dyskinesia.* TD is by definition a late-onset movement disorder produced by antipsychotic medications. Experience to date suggests that clozapine does *not* produce TD. Furthermore, clozapine can sometimes be used effectively to reverse TD caused by other antipsychotics.
- *Seizures.* Clozapine can lower the seizure threshold and precipitate seizures in susceptible individuals, particularly in those with a history of seizure disorders. The risk of seizures with clozapine is increased at dosages greater than 600 mg/day, but seizures can occur at lower dosages, as well. The risk of seizures is also associated with increasing the clozapine dose too rapidly.
- *Neuroleptic malignant syndrome (NMS).* The symptoms of NMS, a rare, toxic reaction to antipsychotics, including clozapine, are severe muscle stiffness, rigidity, elevated body temperature, increased heart rate, high blood pressure, and sweating. NMS can lead to delirium, coma, and death if medical intervention is not provided. Hence, NMS must be recognized early, because it is a medical emergency requiring immediate cessation of the antipsychotic, hospitalization, and intensive medical treatment.
- *Heatstroke.* Antipsychotics, including clozapine, may induce heatstroke, resulting in elevation of body temperature. High body temperature is potentially dangerous if it is not treated and lowered. Heatstroke usually occurs in patients who have prolonged exposure to warm temperatures and become dehydrated. To prevent heatstroke, the patient should drink plenty of fluids and, in hot weather, avoid prolonged exposure to the sun.

USE IN PREGNANCY AND BREAST FEEDING

Clozapine is classified in **Category B** of the U.S. Food and Drug Administration (FDA) Pregnancy Risk Categories. Studies of its use for pregnant women are not available. In animal studies, no fetal abnormalities were reported. Pregnant women, or women who are planning to become pregnant, should not take clozapine, if possible. However, if the risk of not treating poses a greater danger for the mother and child, the benefits of treatment with clozapine may outweigh any unknown risks.

Clozapine passes into breast milk and can cause harm to the infant when ingested. Therefore, women taking clozapine should not breastfeed.

If you have any questions about this handout, please consult your physician.

INFORMATION ABOUT

OLANZAPINE (ZYPREXA)

FOR PATIENTS AND FAMILIES

Olanzapine (Zyprexa) was first marketed in the United States in 1996, primarily for treatment of schizophrenia and schizoaffective disorder. However, olanzapine was also shown to be effective for treating mood disorders, such as bipolar disorder, and received an indication from the U.S. Food and Drug Administration (FDA) for the treatment of acute mania and in maintenance therapy for bipolar disorder. Recent studies suggest that olanzapine may be effective for the treatment of psychotic depression as well.

Olanzapine is a second-generation antipsychotic, a newer class of antipsychotics that have actions different from those of the older, first-generation antipsychotics. Olanzapine, like the other second-generation antipsychotics, is more effective than the older antipsychotics, such as haloperidol, for treating "negative symptoms" of schizophrenia, such as apathy, lack of motivation, flat emotional expression, withdrawal, and depression. Furthermore, second-generation antipsychotics at standard doses rarely cause side effects associated with movement disorders, such as extrapyramidal symptoms (EPS) and tardive dyskinesia (TD). This is a very important distinction between the newer and older antipsychotics.

Olanzapine is available only as the brand Zyprexa, in 2.5-, 5-, 7.5-, 10-, 15-, and 20-mg strength tablets and in rapidly dissolving wafers (Zyprexa-Zydis) that do not need swallowing. Zyprexa is also available in an injectable for for intramuscular administration in acute treatment.

HOW OLANZAPINE IS PRESCRIBED

The usual starting daily dose is 5 mg, and the dosage is increased to a target of 10 mg/day within several days. In acute treatment, a dosage range of 15 to 20 mg/day is usually needed for antipsychotic treatment, although some patients require dosages higher than 20 mg/day. Olanzapine may be taken in divided doses twice a day, but it is preferably taken as a single bedtime dose.

PROPER USE OF YOUR MEDICATION

Storing Your Medication

- Keep your medication in a tamper-resistant vial and out of reach of children.
- Store your medication so that it is kept from excessive heat, moisture, and direct light.
- Keep your medication in its original prescription vial with the label intact to prevent others from taking the medication inadvertently.

Taking Your Medication

- Take your medication as instructed by your physician. Do not abruptly stop taking your medication without consulting your physician.
- If you miss a dose, take it as soon as possible. However, if it is near the time of your next dose, skip the dose you missed and go back to your regular dosing schedule, but do not double-up the dose.
- Olanzapine may be taken with food or at mealtime without affecting its absorption.

Use of Alcohol and Other Medications

Individuals should refrain from alcohol consumption while taking olanzapine. When the two are combined, sedation and drowsiness may be significantly enhanced. Some medications, including over-the-counter medicines, may interact with olanzapine. The drug interaction may *lower* the blood level of the affected drug and decrease the drug's effectiveness; or, it may *elevate* the blood level of the affected drug and induce toxicity. A number of drugs when combined with olanzapine may make certain side effects worse. Inform your doctor of all the prescription and over-the-counter medications you are taking. If you have any questions or concerns about your medications, consult your physician or pharmacist.

POSSIBLE SIDE EFFECTS

- *Sedation.* Olanzapine often produces significant sedation and drowsiness at the start of therapy, but these side effects eventually subside as the patient develops greater tolerance to the medication. Frequently, taking olanzapine in a single bedtime dose can mitigate the patient's daytime drowsiness.

- *Orthostatic hypotension.* Olanzapine may oppose the body's ability to elevate blood pressure in response to a change in position. **Orthostatic hypotension** occurs when blood pressure cannot be raised in time as the person stands up. As a result, the individual feels light-headed and dizzy and may faint and fall. By learning to rise slowly and allowing the blood pressure to adjust gradually, the individual can minimize orthostatic hypotension. This practice is important when standing up after sitting for long periods or when rising from bed. Usually the individual adapts to postural hypotension. If the problem is severe, lowering the dose or switching to another medication may correct it.

- *Dry mouth.* This side effect may be bothersome in the beginning. Often it subsides when the patient develops greater tolerance to the medication. Chewing sugarless gum or sucking on sugarless candy may provide some relief for the patient.

- *Constipation.* Olanzapine may slow gastrointestinal movement and cause constipation. To prevent constipation, the patient should increase fluid intake, increase fiber content in the diet, and exercise regularly. Bulk laxatives or a stool softener, such as docusate, may be needed at times to relieve constipation.

- *Blurred vision.* Olanzapine may cause blurred vision and affect accommodation (ability of the eye to adjust when looking at close objects). If this occurs, the patient should inform his or her physician. Lowering the dose may eliminate this problem.

- *Weight gain.* Weight gain is a common side effect of olanzapine, and some patients may experience significant weight gain from the medication. Weight gain may be due to increased appetite or some underlying metabolic change. The major concern from excessive weight gain is the health consequences to the patient, including the potential for developing diabetes and cardiovascular disease. Furthermore, patients may stop taking their medication when they become self-conscious about excessive weight. If this becomes problematic, the patient should consult with his or her physician. Both the physician and patient can agree on a supervised program to include diet and exercise to reduce and control weight. The alternative is switching to another second-generation antipsychotic medication that may be more weight-neutral.

- *Altered glucose metabolism and diabetes.* Atypical antipsychotics may affect the way the body handles glucose, perhaps by decreasing the body's sensitivity to insulin. As a result, glucose levels in the blood may be elevated (**hyperglycemia**). Cases of drug-induced **diabetes** have been reported with olanzapine and clozapine.

- *Extrapyramidal side effects.* Neurologic side effects from antipsychotic medications resulting in movement disorders are commonly known as **extrapyramidal symptoms** (EPS). EPS include akathisia, Parkinson-like symptoms, and dystonia. Conventional antipsychotic medications such as haloperidol frequently induce EPS, whereas olanzapine, at standard doses, rarely produces EPS.

  At higher doses, some patients may experience **akathisia,** which is described as an inner feeling of restlessness, expressed by constant pacing, inability to sit still, nervousness, and even agitation. Reducing the dose of olanzapine is usually the most effective treatment of akathisia. Also, at higher doses, olanzapine may induce **Parkinson-like symptoms,** which are manifested in movement disorders very similar to **Parkinson's disease.** Patients with Parkinson-like symptoms may have a tremor of the fingers and hands, muscle stiffness, a shuffle when walking, stooped posture, drooling, and a masklike face. These side effects can be effectively treated with an anticholinergic agent like **benztropine** (Cogentin), **diphenhydramine** (Benadryl), or **trihexyphenidyl** (Artane).

Patients should be aware of an EPS that may occur with any antipsychotic medication, although it occurs rarely with olanzapine. This reaction, called **dystonia,** is a sudden spasm of the muscles of the tongue, jaw, or neck. Although it can be very frightening, it is not an allergic reaction. The patient should immediately seek medical attention, because a dystonic reaction can be rapidly reversed with an intramuscular injection of an anticholinergic medication (benztropine or diphenhydramine).

Warning: Olanzapine may cause drowsiness and sedation and impair physical coordination and mental alertness. Until you are sure that these side effects will not impair your ability to perform daily tasks, it is important to avoid potentially dangerous activities, such as driving a car or operating machinery.

POSSIBLE ADVERSE REACTIONS

- *Tardive dyskinesia.* TD is by definition a late-onset abnormal, involuntary movement disorder that commonly includes "pill-rolling" movements of the fingers, darting and writhing movements of the tongue, lip puckering, facial grimacing, and other irregular movements. Experience to date suggests that olanzapine rarely produces TD, but there may be a risk from chronic exposure to antipsychotics. With olanzapine, as with all antipsychotics, routine monitoring for TD is important.

- *Seizures.* Olanzapine may lower the seizure threshold and precipitate seizures in susceptible individuals, particularly those with a history of seizure disorders. The risk of seizures is very low. Olanzapine, however, should be used cautiously in patients with a history of seizures.

- *Neuroleptic malignant syndrome (NMS).* NMS is a rare, toxic reaction to antipsychotics, including olanzapine. The symptoms are severe muscle stiffness, rigidity, elevated body temperature, increased heart rate and blood pressure, irregular pulse, and sweating. NMS can lead to delirium and coma. It may be fatal if medical intervention is not immediately provided. There are no tests that can predict if an individual may be susceptible to developing NMS when treated with an antipsychotic. Hence, NMS must be recognized early because it is a medical emergency that requires immediate discontinuation of the antipsychotic, timely hospitalization, and intensive medical treatment.

- *Heatstroke.* Patients taking antipsychotics may be susceptible to heatstroke when they are exposed to very hot weather and become dehydrated. To prevent heatstroke, the patient should drink plenty of fluids and avoid prolonged exposure in hot weather.

USE IN PREGNANCY AND BREAST FEEDING

Olanzapine is classified in **Category C** of the FDA Pregnancy Risk Categories. There are no clinical studies or available information to use in determining the risk of olanzapine use during pregnancy; therefore, the extent of risk is not known. Women who are pregnant, or who are planning to become pregnant, should not take olanzapine. However, if the risk of not treating poses a greater danger for the mother and child, the benefits from olanzapine may outweigh any unknown risks.

It is not known if olanzapine passes into breast milk. However, it is recommended that women taking olanzapine not breastfeed.

If you have any questions about this handout, please consult your physician.

INFORMATION ABOUT

QUETIAPINE (SEROQUEL)

FOR PATIENTS AND FAMILIES

Quetiapine (Seroquel) is an antipsychotic medication used in the treatment of psychotic disorders, including schizophrenia, schizoaffective disorder, psychotic depression, and acute mania in bipolar disorder. Quetiapine is one of the second-generation antipsychotics, a new class of medicines that have actions different from those of older, first-generation antipsychotics like **chlorpromazine** (Thorazine) and **haloperidol** (Haldol). Second-generation antipsychotics are more effective than the earlier antipsychotics in reducing "negative" symptoms of schizophrenia, such as apathy, lack of motivation, flat emotional expression, and withdrawal and isolation from people. The incidences of neurologic side effects that result in movement disorders are very low with quetiapine, and therefore quetiapine is better tolerated than the older antipsychotics.

Quetiapine is marketed in the United States only as the brand **Seroquel.** Seroquel is available in 25-, 100-, 200-, and 300-mg tablets.

HOW QUETIAPINE IS PRESCRIBED

The usual starting dose is 25 mg twice a day, and the dose is gradually increased in increments of 25 mg once a day, with a target dosage of 400 mg/day by the end of the second week. If needed, the dose may be increased further until therapeutic response is achieved. The dosage may range from 400 to 800 mg/day, taken in divided doses at least twice a day. The maximum daily dose for quetiapine is 800 mg.

PROPER USE OF YOUR MEDICATION

Storing Your Medication

- Keep your medication in a tamper-resistant vial and out of reach of children.
- Store your medication so that it is kept from excessive heat, moisture, and direct light.
- Keep your medication in its original prescription vial with the label intact to prevent others from taking the medication inadvertently.
- Do not use your medication past its expiration date.

Taking Your Medication

- Take your medication as instructed by your physician. Do not abruptly stop taking your medication without consulting your physician. Discontinuation of your medication may result in relapse.
- If you miss a dose, take the dose as soon as possible. However, if it is near the time of your next dose, skip the dose you missed and go back to your regular dosing schedule, but do not double-up the dose.
- Quetiapine may be taken with food or at mealtime without affecting its absorption.

Use of Alcohol and Other Medications

Patients taking quetiapine should refrain from alcohol consumption. Sedation and drowsiness may be exacerbated when alcohol is combined with quetiapine. This may impair judgment, thinking, and coordination and, therefore, the ability to perform tasks. Some medications, including over-the-counter medicines, can adversely interact with quetiapine. The drug interaction may *lower* the blood level of the affected drug and decrease the drug's effectiveness; or, it may *elevate* the blood level of the affected drug and result in toxicity. When certain drugs are combined with quetiapine, they may make some side effects worse. Inform your doctor of all the prescription and over-the-counter medications you are taking. If you have any questions or concerns about your medications, consult your physician or pharmacist.

POSSIBLE SIDE EFFECTS

- *Sedation and drowsiness.* Sedation and drowsiness are the most common complaints from patients taking quetiapine, especially immediately after starting therapy. These side effects eventually subside as the patient develops tolerance to the medication. For most patients, taking a larger portion of the divided dose at bedtime mitigates daytime sedation.
- *Orthostatic hypotension.* Quetiapine may oppose the body's ability to elevate blood pressure in response to a change in position. If the blood pressure cannot elevate in time to compensate for the change in position as the individual rises from a lying or sitting position, **orthostatic hypotension** ensues. As a result, the individual feels light-headed and dizzy, has a rapid heart rate, and may faint and fall. To prevent orthostatic hypotension, after sitting for long periods or when getting out of bed, the patient should rise slowly to allow the blood pressure to adjust gradually. Usually the individual adapts to orthostatic hypotension. If the problem is severe, lowering the dose or switching to another medication may correct this side effect.
- *Constipation.* Quetiapine may slow gastrointestinal movement and cause constipation. To prevent constipation, the patient should increase fluid intake, eat a high-fiber diet, and exercise regularly. A bulk laxative or a stool softener, such as docusate, may be needed at times to relieve constipation.
- *Weight gain.* Although quetiapine does not induce weight gain as much as olanzapine or clozapine, some patients may gain weight from quetiapine. The major concern from excessive weight gain is the health consequences to the patient, including the potential for developing diabetes and cardiovascular disease. Furthermore, patients may stop taking their medication when they become self-conscious about putting on excessive weight. The patient should consult with the physician if gaining weight becomes a problem. Both physician and patient can mutually agree on a supervised program, including diet and exercise, to reduce and control weight. The alternative is to switch to another atypical antipsychotic that may be more weight-neutral.
- *Extrapyramidal side effects.* Neurologic side effects from antipsychotic medications resulting in movement disorders are commonly known as **extrapyramidal symptoms** (EPS). EPS include akathisia, Parkinson-like symptoms, and dystonia. Conventional antipsychotic medications such as haloperidol frequently induce EPS, whereas quetiapine causes fewer EPS side effects.

  At higher doses of quetiapine, patients may experience **akathisia,** which is described as an inner feeling of restlessness, expressed by constant pacing, inability to sit still, nervousness, and even agitation. Reducing the dose of antipsychotic is usually the most effective treatment for akathisia. If reducing the dose is not an option, the physician may add another medication to treat the akathisia. The agent commonly prescribed is **propranolol** (Inderal), which belongs to a class of medicines called **beta-blockers.** Beta-blocking agents have many different uses, but they are primarily used for treating heart disease and hypertension.

  Patients taking higher doses of quetiapine may experience **Parkinson-like symptoms**. Antipsychotic-induced Parkinson-like symptoms are similar to **Parkinson's disease.** Patients may experience tremor of the fingers and hands, muscle stiffness, a shuffle when walking, stooped posture, drooling, and a masklike face. These side effects are reversible and effectively treated with an anticholinergic agent such as **benztropine** (Cogentin), **diphenhydramine** (Benadryl), or **trihexyphenidyl** (Artane).

Dystonia is another type of movement disorder induced by antipsychotics. The incidence of dystonia from quetiapine is very low, but this reaction may occur with any antipsychotic. Dystonia is manifested as a sudden spasm of the muscles of the tongue, jaw, or neck. It is not an allergic reaction, but it can be very frightening for the patient. The patient should immediately seek medical attention, because a dystonic reaction can be rapidly reversed with an intramuscular injection of benztropine or diphenhydramine.

Warning: Quetiapine may cause drowsiness and sedation and impair physical coordination and mental alertness. Until you are sure that these side effects will not impair your ability to perform daily tasks, it is important to avoid potentially dangerous activities, such as driving a car or operating machinery.

POSSIBLE ADVERSE REACTIONS

- *Tardive dyskinesia (TD).* TD is by definition a late-onset abnormal, involuntary movement disorder that commonly includes "pill-rolling" movements of the fingers, darting and writhing movements of the tongue, lip puckering, facial grimacing, and other irregular movements. Current data suggest that the incidence of TD from quetiapine is much lower than that from conventional antipsychotics such as haloperidol. With quetiapine, as with all antipsychotics, routine monitoring for TD is important.
- *Seizures.* Quetiapine may lower the seizure threshold and precipitate seizures in susceptible individuals, particularly those with a history of seizure disorders. However, the risk of seizures is very low. Quetiapine, however, should be used cautiously in patients with a history of seizures.
- *Neuroleptic malignant syndrome (NMS).* NMS is a rare, toxic reaction to all antipsychotics, including quetiapine. The symptoms are severe muscle stiffness, rigidity, elevated body temperature, increased heart rate and blood pressure, irregular pulse, and sweating. NMS can lead to delirium and coma. It may be fatal if medical intervention is not immediately provided. There are no tests that can predict whether an individual is susceptible to developing NMS when exposed to an antipsychotic. Hence, NMS must be recognized early, as it is a medical emergency that requires immediate discontinuation of the antipsychotic, timely hospitalization, and intensive medical treatment.
- *Heatstroke.* Patients taking quetiapine may be susceptible to heatstroke when exposed to very hot weather and become dehydrated. To prevent heatstroke, the patient should drink plenty of fluids and avoid prolonged exposure to hot weather.

USE IN PREGNANCY AND BREAST FEEDING

Quetiapine is classified in **Category C** of the U.S. Food and Drug Administration's (FDA) Pregnancy Risk Categories. There are no studies or available information to determine the risk of using quetiapine during pregnancy. The extent of risk to the fetus is not known. Women who are pregnant, or who are planning to become pregnant, should not take quetiapine. However, if the risk of not treating poses a greater danger for the mother and child, the benefits from quetiapine may outweigh any unknown risks.

It is not known if quetiapine passes into human breast milk. It is recommended that women taking quetiapine not breastfeed.

If you have any questions about this handout, please consult your physician.

Information About

Risperidone (Risperdal and Risperdal Consta)

for Patients and Families

Risperidone (Risperdal) is an antipsychotic medication used in the treatment of psychotic disorders, including schizophrenia, schizoaffective disorder and psychotic depression, and acute mania in bipolar disorder. Risperidone is a second-generation antipsychotic, a new class of medicines that have actions different from those of the older, first-generation antipsychotics such as haloperidol. Risperidone, as well as the other second-generation antipsychotics, are more effective than the older antipsychotics, such as haloperidol, for treating "negative" symptoms of schizophrenia, such as apathy, lack of motivation, flat emotional expression, withdrawal, and depression. Furthermore, the second-generation antipsychotics at standard doses rarely cause side effects associated with movement disorders, such as extrapyramidal symptoms (EPS) and tardive dyskinesia (TD). This is a very important distinction between the atypical and typical antipsychotics.

Risperidone is marketed in the United States only as the brand Risperdal. It is available as tablets in 0.25-, 0.5-, 1- 2-, 3-, and 4-mg strengths. Risperdal also comes in an oral solution, in a concentration of 1 mg/mL, as well as in rapidly dissolving tablets (Risperdal M-Tab) that do not require swallowing. A long-acting, intramuscular injection of risperidone (Risperdal Consta) was introduced recently, providing patients another dosing option, especially those who cannot adhere to taking the oral medication every day.

Risperdal Consta is administered every 2 weeks by intramuscular injection. For patients who have never taken risperidone, a trial is recommended to establish tolerability to oral Risperdal. The recommended starting dose is 25 mg every 2 weeks. Generally, it takes about 3 weeks for Risperdal Consta to achieve therapeutic blood levels, and the patient should continue taking oral Risperdal (or another antipsychotic) with the first injection. The oral antipsychotic may be discontinued after 3 weeks, before the second injection. Thereafter, the patient is maintained on an injection schedule every 2 weeks. Most patients respond to 25 mg, but some may benefit from a higher dose of 37.5 mg or 50 mg. The dose, however, should not exceed 50 mg every 2 weeks.

HOW RISPERIDONE IS PRESCRIBED

The usual starting dose is 0.5–1 mg twice a day in the first week, and the dose is then increased to 1–2 mg twice a day in the second week. If needed, the dose may be increased in the third week to 2–3 mg twice a day. The usual target dosage is 4–6 mg/day. Some patients may require a dosage greater than 6 mg/day, but the dosage should not exceed 8 mg/day. Generally, side effects from risperidone may be minimized when the dose is increased slowly.

PROPER USE OF YOUR MEDICATION

Storing Your Medication

- Keep your medication in a tamper-resistant vial and out of reach of children.
- Store your medication so that it is kept from excessive heat, moisture, and direct light.
- Keep your medication in its original prescription vial with the label intact to prevent others from taking the medication inadvertently.
- Do not use your medication past the expiration date found on the prescription label.

Taking Your Medication

- Take your medication as instructed by your physician. Do not abruptly stop taking your medication without consulting your physician.
- If you miss a dose, take it as soon as possible. However, if it is near to the time of your next dose, skip the dose you missed and go back to your regular dosing schedule, but do not double-up the dose.
- Risperidone may be taken with food without affecting its absorption.
- If you are taking Risperdal Oral Solution, be sure to use the dispensing pipette that comes with your prescription. It is calibrated in milligrams (mg) and milliliters (mL) for ease of measuring a dose. Simply pull the plunger up to the calibrated mark (mg or mL) to the measured dose. Risperidone solution may be mixed with a small amount of water before it is taken.

Use of Alcohol and Other Medications

Individuals should refrain from using alcohol while taking risperidone. When alcohol is combined with risperidone, sedation and drowsiness may become significantly worse. Some medications, including over-the-counter medicines, may adversely interact with risperidone. The drug interaction may *lower* the blood level of the affected drug and decrease the drug's effectiveness; or, it may *elevate* the blood level of the affected drug and result in toxicity. When a number of drugs are combined with risperidone, they may make some side effects worse. Inform your physician of all the prescription and over-the-counter medications you are taking. If you have any questions or concerns about your medications, consult your physician or pharmacist.

POSSIBLE SIDE EFFECTS

- *Sedation.* Risperidone often produces sedation and drowsiness at the start of therapy, but as the patient develops tolerance to the medication, these side effects subside. Taking risperidone in a single bedtime dose may mitigate daytime sedation.
- *Orthostatic hypotension.* Infrequently, risperidone may oppose the body's ability to elevate blood pressure in response to a change in position. If the blood pressure cannot elevate in time to compensate for the change in position as the individual rises from a lying or sitting position, **orthostatic hypotension** ensues. As a result, the individual feels light-headed and dizzy, has a rapid heart rate, and may faint and fall. By learning to rise slowly to allow the blood pressure to adjust gradually, the individual may minimize orthostatic hypotension. This practice is important when standing up after sitting for long periods or when rising from bed. Usually the individual adapts to postural hypotension. If the problem is severe, lowering the dose or switching to another medication may correct this side effect.
- *Constipation.* Risperidone may slow gastrointestinal movement and result in constipation. To prevent constipation, the patient should increase fluid intake, eat a high-fiber diet, and exercise regularly. A bulk laxative, such as Metamucil, or a stool softener, such as docusate, may be needed at times to relieve constipation.
- *Weight gain.* Risperidone does not induce as much weight gain as olanzapine or clozapine. However, some patients may experience weight gain from risperidone. The major concern from excessive weight is the health consequences to the patient, including the potential for developing diabetes and cardiovascular disease. Furthermore, some patients may stop taking their medication when they become self-conscious about putting on excessive weight. The patient should consult with the physician if gaining weight becomes a problem. Both physician and patient can mutually agree on a supervised program, including diet and exercise, to reduce and control weight. If this does not work, the next alternative is to switch to another atypical antipsychotic medication that will not induce weight gain.
- *Extrapyramidal side effects.* Neurologic side effects from antipsychotic medications resulting in movement disorders are commonly known as **extrapyramidal symptoms** (EPS). EPS include akathisia, Parkinson-like symptoms, and dystonia. Conventional antipsychotic medications such as haloperidol frequently induce EPS, whereas risperidone, at lower doses, produces fewer EPS. Risperidone may induce side effects that mimic **Parkinson's disease.** Patients with **Parkinson-like symptoms** may have a tremor of the fingers and hands, muscle stiffness, a shuffle when walking, stooped posture, drooling, and a masklike face. These side effects can be effectively treated with an anticholinergic agent such as **benztropine** (Cogentin), **diphenhydramine** (Benadryl), or **trihexyphenidyl** (Artane).

132

At higher doses, some patients may experience **akathisia** from risperidone, which is described as an inner feeling of restlessness, expressed by constant pacing, inability to sit still, nervousness, and even agitation. Reducing the dose of risperidone is usually the most effective treatment for akathisia. If reducing the dose is not an option, the physician may add another medication to treat the akathisia. The agent commonly prescribed is **propranolol** (Inderal), which belongs to a class of medicines called **beta-blockers.** Beta-blocking agents are primarily used for treating heart disease and hypertension, but they have many other uses as well.

Dystonia is another type of movement disorder induced by antipsychotics, although it infrequently occurs with risperidone. This reaction is manifested as a sudden spasm of the muscles of the tongue, jaw, or neck. It can be very frightening for the patient, but it is not an allergic reaction. The patient should immediately seek medical attention, because a dystonic reaction may be rapidly reversed with an intramuscular injection of an anticholinergic medication such as benztropine or diphenhydramine.

- *Prolactin elevation.* Risperidone may affect an area of the brain known as the **hypothalamus** and cause elevation of a hormone called **prolactin.** Prolactin stimulates the mammary glands in females, as well as in males. When elevated, prolactin may cause breast enlargement and milk secretion in both women and men. Elevated prolactin levels may play a role in irregular or lack of menses in women and may cause impotence in men.

- *Other possible side effects.* Increased pulse, insomnia, nausea, and stuffy nose are other possible side effects that may be experienced while taking risperidone.

> **Warning:** Risperidone may cause drowsiness and sedation and impair physical coordination and mental alertness. Until you are sure that these side effects will not impair your ability to perform daily tasks, it is important to avoid potentially dangerous activities, such as driving a car or operating machinery.

POSSIBLE ADVERSE REACTIONS

- *Tardive dyskinesia (TD).* TD is by definition a late-onset abnormal, involuntary movement disorder that commonly includes "pill-rolling" movements of the fingers, darting and writhing movements of the tongue, lip puckering, facial grimacing, and other irregular movements. Current data suggest that the incidence of TD from risperidone is rare. With risperidone, as with all antipsychotics, routine monitoring for TD is important.

- *Seizures.* Risperidone can lower the seizure threshold and precipitate seizures in susceptible individuals, particularly those with a history of seizure disorders. The risk of seizures is very low. However, risperidone should be used cautiously in patients with a history of seizures.

- *Neuroleptic malignant syndrome (NMS).* NMS is a rare, toxic reaction to antipsychotics, including risperidone. The symptoms are severe muscle stiffness, rigidity, elevated body temperature, increased heart rate and blood pressure, irregular pulse, and sweating. NMS can lead to delirium and coma. It may be fatal if medical intervention is not immediately provided. There are no tests that can predict whether an individual is susceptible to developing NMS when treated with an antipsychotic. Hence, NMS must be recognized early because it is a medical emergency that requires immediate discontinuation of the antipsychotic, hospitalization, and intensive medical treatment.

- *Heatstroke.* Patients taking risperidone may be susceptible to heatstroke when exposed to very hot weather and become dehydrated. To prevent heatstroke, the patient should drink plenty of fluids and avoid prolong exposure in hot weather.

USE IN PREGNANCY AND BREAST FEEDING

Risperidone is classified in **Category C** of the U.S. Food and Drug Administration (FDA) Pregnancy Risk Categories. There are no studies or available information to determine the risk of using risperidone during pregnancy. The extent of risk to the fetus is not known. Women who are pregnant, or who are planning to become pregnant, should not take risperidone. However, if the risk of not treating poses a greater danger for the mother and child, the benefits of treatment with risperidone may outweigh any unknown risks.

Risperidone may also pass into human breast milk, but it is not known to what extent. Therefore, women taking risperidone should not breastfeed because it may have harmful effects on the infant when ingested.

If you have any questions about this handout, please consult your physician.

INFORMATION ABOUT

ZIPRASIDONE (GEODON)

FOR PATIENTS AND FAMILIES

Ziprasidone (Geodon) is an antipsychotic medication used in the treatment of psychotic disorders, including schizophrenia, schizoaffective disorder and psychotic depression, and acute mania in bipolar disorder. Ziprasidone is a second-generation antipsychotic, a new class of medicines with actions different from those of the older, first-generation antipsychotics such as **chlorpromazine** (Thorazine) and **haloperidol** (Haldol). The second-generation antipsychotics are more effective than the older antipsychotics in reducing the "negative" symptoms of schizophrenia, such as apathy, lack of motivation, flat emotional expression, depression, and withdrawal and isolation from people. Furthermore, second-generation antipsychotics at standard doses rarely cause side effects associated with movement disorders, such as extrapyramidal symptoms (EPS) and tardive dyskinesia (TD). This is a very important distinction between the newer and older antipsychotics.

Ziprasidone is marketed under the brand name **Geodon.** Geodon is available in 20-, 40-, 60-, and 80-mg capsules. It also comes in a short-acting injectable form for acute treatment.

HOW ZIPRASIDONE IS PRESCRIBED

The recommended starting dose is 20–40 mg twice a day taken with food. The dose is adjusted on the basis of individual response. The effective dosage range is usually between 60 and 80 mg twice a day (120–160 mg/day).

PROPER USE OF YOUR MEDICATION

Storing Your Medication

- Keep your medication in a tamper-resistant vial and out of reach of children.
- Store your medication so that it is kept from excessive heat, moisture, and direct light.
- Keep your medication in its original prescription vial with the label intact to prevent others from taking the medication inadvertently.

Taking Your Medication

- Take your medication as instructed by your physician. Do not abruptly stop taking your medication without telling your physician. Discontinuation of your medication may result in relapse.
- If you miss a dose, take it as soon as possible. However, if it is near the time of your next dose, skip the dose you missed and go back to your regular dosing schedule, but do not double-up the dose.
- Ziprasidone may be taken with or without food. If it upsets your stomach, take it at mealtime.

Use of Alcohol and Other Medications

Individuals should refrain from using alcohol while taking ziprasidone. When alcohol is combined with ziprasidone, sedation and drowsiness, common side effects of the medication, may be made significantly worse. This may impair judgment, the ability to think clearly, and coordination and, therefore, the ability to perform tasks. Some medications, including over-the-counter medicines, may interact with ziprasidone. The drug interaction may *lower* the blood level of the affected drug and decrease the drug's effectiveness; or, it may *elevate* the blood level of the affected drug and result in toxicity. When certain drugs are combined with ziprasidone, they may make some side effects worse. Inform your doctor of all the prescription and over-the-counter medications you are taking. If you have any questions or concerns about your medications, consult your physician or pharmacist.

POSSIBLE SIDE EFFECTS

- *Sedation and drowsiness.* Sedation and drowsiness are the most common complaints expressed by patients taking ziprasidone, especially immediately after starting therapy. These side effects eventually subside as the patient develops tolerance to the medication.

- *Orthostatic hypotension.* Ziprasidone may oppose the body's ability to elevate blood pressure in response to a change in position. If the blood pressure cannot elevate in time to compensate for the change in position as the individual rises from a lying or sitting position, **orthostatic hypotension** ensues. As a result, the individual feels light-headed and dizzy, has a rapid heart rate, and may faint and fall. To prevent orthostatic hypotension after sitting for long periods or when getting out of bed, the patient should rise slowly to allow the blood pressure to adjust gradually. Orthostatic hypotension from ziprasidone is generally mild, and the patient can usually adapt to it after the first or second week of therapy. If the problem is severe, however, the physician may lower the dose or switch to another medication to correct this side effect.

- *Gastrointestinal side effects.* Dry mouth, nausea, vomiting, constipation, diarrhea, abdominal cramping, and pain are some of the gastrointestinal side effects experienced by patients taking ziprasidone, especially at the onset of therapy. These side effects are usually mild and become less bothersome as the patient develops tolerance to them.

- *Weight gain.* Ziprasidone induces very little weight gain as compared with other antipsychotics such as clozapine and olanzapine. However, some patients may experience weight gain from the ziprasidone. The patient should consult with the physician if excessive weight gain becomes a problem.

- *Extrapyramidal side effects.* Antipsychotic-induced neurologic side effects that cause movement disorders are commonly known as **extrapyramidal symptoms** (EPS). EPS include akathisia, Parkinson-like symptoms, and dystonia. Conventional antipsychotic medications such as like haloperidol frequently induce EPS. Ziprasidone, on the other hand, rarely induces EPS, and when present, the symptoms generally occur at higher doses.

  Some patients may experience **akathisia** from ziprasidone, which is described as an inner feeling of restlessness, expressed by constant pacing, inability to sit still, nervousness, and even agitation. Reducing the dose of antipsychotic is usually the most effective treatment of akathisia. If reducing the dose is not an option, the physician may add another medication to treat the akathisia. The agent commonly prescribed is **propranolol** (Inderal), which belongs to a class of medicines called **beta-blockers.** Beta-blocking agents have many different uses, but they are primarily used for treating heart disease and hypertension.

  Parkinson-like symptoms are other possible EPS side effects from ziprasidone. Antipsychotic-induced Parkinson-like symptoms are similar to **Parkinson's disease.** Patients with Parkinson-like symptoms may experience a tremor of the fingers and hands, muscle stiffness, a shuffle when walking, stooped posture, drooling, and a masklike face. These side effects are reversible and effectively treated with an anticholinergic agent such as **benztropine** (Cogentin), **diphenhydramine** (Benadryl), or **trihexyphenidyl** (Artane).

  Dystonia is another type of movement disorder induced by antipsychotics, although it rarely occurs with ziprasidone. However, as with all antipsychotics, there is the potential for dystonia with ziprasidone. This reaction is manifested by a sudden spasm of the muscles of the tongue, jaw, or neck. It is not an allergic reaction, but it can be very frightening for the patient. The patient should immediately seek medical attention, because a dystonic reaction can be rapidly reversed with an intramuscular injection of benztropine or diphenhydramine.

- *Other possible side effects.* Headache, stuffy nose, and skin rash are other possible side effects with ziprasidone.

Warning: Ziprasidone may cause drowsiness and sedation and impair physical coordination and mental alertness. Until you are sure that these side effects will not impair your ability to perform daily tasks, it is important to avoid potentially dangerous activities, such as driving a car or operating machinery.

POSSIBLE ADVERSE REACTIONS

- *Prolongation of electrical conduction.* Ziprasidone may impair electrical conduction of the heart. On an electrocardiogram (ECG), this impairment may show up as a prolonged interval (QT), a segment on the ECG graph, in the conduction cycle. This type of prolongation may be associated with arrhythmias, which are irregular heartbeats due to abnormal electrical conduction. Current data, however, show ziprasidone to be quite safe. The risk of developing arrhythmia from ziprasidone is very low. The risk, however, may be increased if the patient has a history of conduction defect or cardiac arrhythmia. Moreover, some drugs that prolong QT interval, when combined with ziprasidone, may potentiate the risk of arrhythmias. Therefore, your physician will determine if ziprasidone is safe for you and may order ECGs to monitor the medication therapy.

- *Tardive dyskinesia.* TD is by definition a late-onset abnormal, involuntary movement disorder. It is potentially an irreversible condition with symptoms that commonly include "pill-rolling" movements of the fingers, darting and writhing movements of the tongue, lip puckering, facial grimacing, and other irregular movements. From experience with conventional antipsychotics, it has been suggested that the risk of developing TD is associated with the duration and amount of antipsychotics the patient was exposed to over the life of treatment. As the duration and amount of exposure to antipsychotics increase, so does the patient's risk of developing TD. However, the incidence of TD from atypical antipsychotics is much lower than from conventional antipsychotics. Because ziprasidone was just recently introduced to the United States, current data about the drug's potential for causing TD are limited. The risk of developing TD from ziprasidone is expected to be low. As with all antipsychotics, routine monitoring for TD is important.

- *Seizures.* Ziprasidone may lower the seizure threshold and precipitate seizures in susceptible individuals, particularly those with a history of seizure disorders. The risk of seizures is very low, however. Ziprasidone should be prescribed cautiously in patients with a history of seizures.

- *Neuroleptic malignant syndrome (NMS).* NMS is a rare, toxic reaction to antipsychotics, including ziprasidone. The symptoms are severe muscle stiffness, rigidity, elevated body temperature, increased heart rate and blood pressure, irregular pulse, and sweating. NMS can lead to delirium and coma. It may be fatal if medical intervention is not provided promptly. There are no tests that can predict whether an individual is susceptible to developing NMS when exposed to an antipsychotic. Hence, NMS must be recognized early, because it is a medical emergency that requires immediate discontinuation of the antipsychotic, timely hospitalization, and intensive medical treatment.

- *Heatstroke.* Patients taking ziprasidone may be susceptible to heatstroke when exposed to very hot weather and become dehydrated. To prevent heatstroke, the patient should drink plenty of fluids and avoid prolong exposure in hot weather.

USE IN PREGNANCY AND BREAST FEEDING

Ziprasidone is classified in **Category C** of the U.S. Food and Drug Administration (FDA) Pregnancy Risk Categories. There are no studies or adequate information to determine the extent of risk of aripiprazole during pregnancy. The risk to the fetus is unknown. In animal studies, however, some fetal abnormalities were found after maternal exposure to ziprasidone. Interpretation of these animal studies in regarding to human risk is unclear. Women who are pregnant, or who are planning to become pregnant, should not take ziprasidone. However, if the risk of not treating poses a greater danger for the mother and child, the benefits of treatment with ziprasidone may outweigh any unknown risks.

It is not known whether ziprasidone is excreted into human breast milk. It is recommended that women taking ziprasidone not breastfeed. Ziprasidone may have harmful effects on the infant if ingested.

If you have any questions about this handout, please consult your physician.

INFORMATION ABOUT

THE FIRST-GENERATION ANTIPSYCHOTICS

FOR PATIENTS AND FAMILIES

- ○ **Chlorpromazine (Thorazine)**
- ○ **Fluphenazine (Prolixin)**
- ○ **Haloperidol (Haldol)**
- ○ **Loxapine (Loxitane)**
- ○ **Mesoridazine (Serentil)**
- ○ **Trifluoperazine (Stelazine)**

- ○ **Molindone (Moban)**
- ○ **Perphenazine (Trilafon)**
- ○ **Pimozide (Orap)**
- ○ **Thioridazine (Mellaril)**
- ○ **Thiothixene (Navane)**

For decades, older, first-generation antipsychotics were the standard of treatment for psychotic disorders. These antipsychotics are also commonly called conventional or *typical* antipsychotics because they differ from the newer, second-generation, *atypical* antipsychotics. The first-generation antipsychotics are also referred to as *neuroleptics* because they induce neurologic side effects.

The first-generation antipsychotics are discussed together as a group in this handout. The second-generation antipsychotics are each discussed separately in individual handouts. Although there are differences between the first-generation antipsychotics, they are similar in many respects in their action and side effects, and so it is simpler to discuss them as a group.

There are 11 first-generation and 6 second-generation antipsychotics available in United States. Of the first-generation antipsychotic agents, haloperidol (Haldol) is the most frequently prescribed.

The first-generation antipsychotics vary in potency. For example, to attain the same effect, it is necessary to take more of a lower-potency agent than of a higher-potency one. The low-potency agents are chlorpromazine (Thorazine), mesoridazine (Serentil), and thioridazine (Mellaril); fluphenazine (Prolixin), haloperidol (Haldol), pimozide (Orap), thiothixene (Navane), and trifluoperazine (Stelazine) are high-potency antipsychotics. The intermediate-potency antipsychotics are loxapine (Loxitane), molindone (Moban), and perphenazine (Trilafon).

How do antipsychotics work? It is not known exactly how antipsychotics work in an organ as complex as the brain. However, the findings support that psychosis may be due to excessive activity of a neurotransmitter in certain areas of the brain. The neurotransmitter in question has been shown to be **dopamine**. Excessive activity of dopamine may be responsible for the overt symptoms of psychosis. Psychosis may be induced with dopamine-enhancing drugs like amphetamine. Antipsychotics exert their action by inhibiting the action of dopamine and thereby reducing psychotic symptoms. Antipsychotics may control the symptoms but do not alter the cause of the illness.

HOW ANTIPSYCHOTICS ARE PRESCRIBED

Antipsychotics are prescribed for treating psychosis in a number of psychiatric disorders, including schizophrenia, schizoaffective disorder, bipolar disorder, psychotic depression, and drug-induced psychosis. Antipsychotics are also used to treat severe obsessive-compulsive disorder, Tourette's disorder, and dementia with agitation.

Physicians may select an antipsychotic on the basis of the patient's past response to other antipsychotics, the side-effect profile of the antipsychotic, and the best match of the patient's symptoms with the antipsychotic. Generally, on an outpatient basis, physicians start patients with a low dose of antipsychotic and then increase the dose gradually to minimize side effects. However, with acutely psychotic patients in the hospital, dosages may be higher and increases in dosage may be more rapid than in an outpatient setting. Frequently, short-acting injectable and oral solution antipsychotics are used in acute treatment.

It is important to understand that antipsychotics act slowly. Although there are some patients who show dramatic, rapid response, the majority of patients improve more slowly, and some may not respond at all. On average, most patients improve and see reduction in symptoms in the first and sixth weeks of therapy. Thereafter, residual symptoms improve more modestly over the next 13 weeks, with little change after week 26. When given enough time, patients may see greater improvement from their medications.

How Long Must Antipsychotics Be Taken?

The duration of treatment depends on the disorder. In drug-induced psychosis, for example, when symptoms are successfully controlled with an antipsychotic, the patient may no longer need the medication as long as there are no residual symptoms. In bipolar disorder, antipsychotics may be administered during the acute phase of mania and discontinued when the manic phase resolves. However, in primary psychotic disorders, such as schizophrenia and schizoaffective disorder, patients may need to continue taking antipsychotics chronically to stay in remission (symptom-free).

PROPER USE OF YOUR MEDICATION

Storing Your Medication

- Keep your medication in a tamper-resistant vial away from the reach of children.
- Store your medication so that it is kept from excessive heat, moisture, and direct sunlight.
- Keep the medication in its original prescription vial with the prescription label intact to prevent others from taking the medication inadvertently.
- Do not use the medication past the expiration date on the prescription label.

Use of Alcohol and Other Medications

It is recommended that individuals taking antipsychotics not consume alcohol. It is important to keep in mind that alcohol is a depressant. Alcohol consumption, especially in excessive amounts, may oppose the action of the medication and exacerbate the patient's illness. Alcohol may exacerbate the side effects from antipsychotics, especially sedation and drowsiness.

There are certain medications that can interact with antipsychotics, particularly drugs that compete for metabolism in the liver. Inform your physician of all the medications you are taking, including over-the-counter medications. If you have any questions or concerns with your medications, consult your physician or pharmacist.

COMMON SIDE EFFECTS

Antipsychotics, like all medications, may cause unwanted side effects. Some are more bothersome than others. Usually patients develop tolerance to mild side effects. However, if side effects are intolerable, decreasing the dose or adding a prophylactic medication may be needed. The alternative is to switch to another antipsychotic medication more compatible for the patient. The more frequent side effects from typical antipsychotics are discussed below.

- *Sedation and fatigue.* Sedation is a very common experience during early treatment, and often patients complain of feeling tired as well. All antipsychotics can be sedating, but low-potency typical antipsychotics, such as chlorpromazine, are the most sedating, whereas high-potency agents, such as haloperidol, are the least.

- *Abnormal movement disorders.* Typical antipsychotics, especially the high-potency agents, can induce movements that mimic **Parkinson's disease.** They cause **Parkinson-like symptoms** that include muscle stiffness, rigidity, tremor, drooling, and a masklike face. The Parkinson-like symptoms and other types of involuntary movements are referred to as **extrapyramidal symptoms** (EPS). EPS may be treated and prevented with antiparkinsonian medications (also called anticholinergic agents), including **benztropine** (Cogentin), **diphenhydramine** (Benadryl), **trihexylphenidyl** (Artane), and **procyclidine** (Kemadrin).

  Dystonia, which occurs shortly after the patient starts an antipsychotic medication, is another form of EPS. It is often manifested by a sudden spasm of the tongue, jaw, and neck. It is not an allergic reaction to the antipsychotic medication. Although a dystonic reaction may be painful and frightening, it can be rapidly reversed with an injection of an anticholinergic medication, such as benztropine or diphenhydramine. With a dystonic reaction, the patient should immediately seek medical attention.

  Akathisia, another form of EPS, is a subjective feeling of restlessness caused by antipsychotics. It is described as a feeling of nervousness (with the need to pace and the inability to sit still), muscular discomfort, and agitation. Akathisia responds poorly to anticholinergic medications. Reduction of the antipsychotic dose is the common approach to treating akathisia. However, use of **propranolol** (Inderal) may be helpful for some patients with akathisia.

- *Orthostatic hypotension.* Antipsychotics, especially the low-potency agents, oppose the body's ability to raise blood pressure when there is a change in position. If the blood pressure cannot elevate in time to compensate for the change in position as the individual rises from a lying or sitting position, **orthostatic hypotension** ensues. As a result, the individual feels light-headed and dizzy, has a rapid heart rate, and may faint and fall. By learning to rise slowly and allow the blood pressure to adjust, the individual may avoid or minimize postural hypotension. This practice is especially important when getting up from a chair after sitting for some time or when rising from bed. Usually the individual adapts to postural hypotension. If the problem is severe, lowering the dose or switching to another medication may correct it.

- *Constipation.* Many antipsychotics may cause constipation. To prevent and treat constipation, the patient should increase fluid intake, eat a high-fiber diet, and increase exercise. Constipation may be aided by use of a bulk laxative, such as Metamucil, or a stool softener, such as docusate. Constipation may be more frequent when anticholinergic and antipsychotic medications are taken concomitantly.

- *Dry mouth.* This side effect is more frequent with low-potency antipsychotics and with anticholinergic medications. Usually when the patient hasd had his or her antipsychotic medication stabilized, the dry mouth subsides. When it persists, unfortunately, reducing the dose of the antipsychotic usually does not reduce this side effect. The individual may get some relief by sucking on sugarless candy or chewing sugarless gum to increase the flow of saliva.

- *Eye problems.* Antipsychotics, especially with the low-potency agents and the combination of anticholinergic medications, may produce **blurred vision** and interference of **accommodation** (failure of the eye to focus when looking at nearby objects). If eye problems occur, contact your physician.

- *Photosensitivity.* The typical antipsychotics, particularly the low-potency antipsychotics such as chlorpromazine, may sensitize the skin (**photosensitivity**) and increase susceptibility to sunburn. To prevent sunburn, it is recommended that the patient use a high-numbered sunscreen and avoid prolonged exposure to direct sunlight.

- *Skin rash.* Skin rash also appears to be more frequent with the low-potency antipsychotics, especially chlorpromazine. If a skin rash develops, it may be indicative of an allergic reaction to the medication. Contact your physician, because the antipsychotic may need to be discontinued.

- *Urinary retention.* Antipsychotics, especially low-potency agents, and anticholinergic medications such as **benztropine** (Cogentin) and **trihexyphenidyl** (Artane) may cause urinary problems because of their effects on the bladder. Urinary retention may be due to decreased flow of urine and may cause difficulty and hesitation on urination. Inform your physician when urinary problems occur.

- *Weight gain.* This is a common side effect with antipsychotic medications. Dietary control and an exercise program may stabilize the patient's weight. If the weight gain cannot be controlled, the alternative is to switch the patient to an antipsychotic with a lower tendency to induce weight gain.

- *Prolactin elevation.* The conventional antipsychotics affect an area of the brain known as the **hypothalamus** and may cause elevation of a hormone called **prolactin**. Prolactin stimulates the mammary glands in females as well as in males. When elevated, prolactin may cause breast enlargement and milk secretion in both women and men. Elevated prolactin levels may play a role in irregular or lack of menses in women and may cause impotence in men.

- *Sexual dysfunction.* Conventional antipsychotics may cause sexual dysfunction by decreasing sex drive (libido); women may lose their ability to achieve orgasm; and men may have difficulty with erection or delayed ejaculation. Patients should not hesitant to discuss any sexual dysfunction with their physician.

POSSIBLE ADVERSE REACTIONS

- *Tardive dyskinesia (TD).* One of the most worrisome side effects of the conventional antipsychotics is TD. Although it can occur early on, TD is by definition a late-onset movement disorder that results from treatment with antipsychotics. The movements usually involve the mouth, tongue, or extremities and are involuntary and repetitive. Apparently, a higher incidence of TD is associated with age, women, and cumulative doses and length of treatment with antipsychotic medication. With early detection of tardive dyskinesia, the patient may be switched to an atypical antipsychotic, such as clozapine, which rarely causes movement disorders.

- *Seizures.* Antipsychotics may lower the seizure threshold and precipitate seizures in susceptible individuals. Low-potency antipsychotics, such as chlorpromazine, appear to cause seizures more often than do other antipsychotics. For patients with a history of seizures, antipsychotics must be carefully monitored.

- *Neuroleptic malignant syndrome (NMS).* NMS is a rare, toxic reaction to antipsychotics. The symptoms of NMS may include severe muscle stiffness, rigidity, elevated body temperature, rapid heart rate, elevated blood pressure, and sweating. NMS can lead to delirium and coma and may be fatal if medical intervention is not immediate. Hence, NMS must be recognized early, because it is a medical emergency that requires immediate cessation of the antipsychotic, timely hospitalization, and intensive medical treatment.

- *Heatstroke.* Patients taking antipsychotics may be susceptible to heatstroke when exposed to very hot weather and become dehydrated. To prevent heatstroke, the patient should drink plenty of fluids and avoid prolong exposure in hot weather.

- *Liver function impairment.* Antipsychotics may impair normal liver function. Generally, the reaction is transient and the patient does not have any symptoms, except mild elevation of liver enzymes. The reaction is reversible and not associated with any permanent liver damage. In more serious reactions, the clinical picture is similar to hepatitis. Symptoms of liver dysfunction include tiredness, flu-like symptoms, yellowing of the skin, particularly the whites of the eyes, and marked elevation of liver enzymes. Because of the possibility of liver impairment, physicians may order blood tests periodically to monitor liver function.

USE IN PREGNANCY AND BREAST FEEDING

All the typical antipsychotics listed previously in this handout are classified in **Category C** in the U.S. Food and Drug Administration (FDA) Pregnancy Risk Categories. They are given this classification because there are no clinical studies on these antipsychotics in women, or there is inadequate information, to determine the risk during pregnancy. Animal studies have found some abnormalities in the fetus during maternal exposure to some of these antipsychotics. However, interpretation of animal studies in regard to human risks is unclear. The risk of typical antipsychotics cannot be ruled out, and a typical antipsychotic should be prescribed during pregnancy only if the benefits outweigh the potential risk.

Chlorpromazine and haloperidol have been detected in breast milk, but it is not known whether the other antipsychotics are excreted in breast milk. Women taking antipsychotic medications should not breastfeed.

If you have any questions about this handout, please consult your physician.

INFORMATION ABOUT

HALOPERIDOL DECANOATE (HALDOL DECANOATE) AND FLUPHENAZINE DECANOATE (PROLIXIN DECANOATE)

FOR PATIENTS AND FAMILIES

Haloperidol decanoate (Haldol Decanoate Injection) and **fluphenazine decanoate** (Prolixin Decanoate Injection) are long-acting injections of the antipsychotics **haloperidol** (Haldol) and **fluphenazine** (Prolixin). In the decanoate formulation, the antipsychotics are suspended in sterile sesame oil to extend the duration of action. The antipsychotic action of the decanoates, however, is not different from that of the oral forms, with the exception of duration of action. The effects of fluphenazine decanoate and haloperidol decanoate can last up to 3 and 4 weeks, respectively.

Both haloperidol and fluphenazine are older, first-generation, high-potency antipsychotics for treating schizophrenia, schizoaffective disorder, psychotic depression, and acute mania in bipolar disorder. A new class of second-generation antipsychotics, such as olanzapine (Zyprexa) and risperidone (Risperdal), has distinct differences and advantages over the older, first-generation agents. Risperidone is also available in a long-acting formulation for injection. When haloperidol decanoate or fluphenazine decanoate is given by intramuscular injection, the drug is "deposited" at the injection site. It is slowly absorbed from the muscle tissues and distributed throughout the body and to the brain, the target organ, where it exerts its antipsychotic effect.

Haloperidol decanoate and fluphenazine decanoate injections are marketed under the trade names **Haldol Decanoate Injection** and **Prolixin Decanoate Injection**. Both drugs are available in generic preparations by various manufacturers. Haloperidol decanoate injection comes in concentrations of 50 mg/mL and 100 mg/mL, whereas fluphenazine decanoate injection comes only in a concentration of 25 mg/mL. (*Note:* The strengths of the decanoates are not equivalent to the strengths of their oral forms on a milligram-per-milligram basis.)

HOW THE DECANOATES ARE PRESCRIBED

The patient, of course, must agree and cooperate with treatment, which requires routine clinic or office visits to receive maintenance injections of the medication. For the patient who cannot adhere to taking daily oral medications, a decanoate antipsychotic may help prevent psychotic relapse due to ongoing problems with noncompliance. Routine maintenance with haloperidol or fluphenazine decanoate ensures that the patient is receiving the medication and the physician is aware when an injection is missed.

Before receiving haloperidol or fluphenazine decanoate, the patient is treated with the short-acting form to determine response and therapeutic dosage. The dosage is usually determined by taking the patient's total daily oral dose of haloperidol or fluphenazine and using a conversion ratio to calculate the decanoate dosage. The dosage, however, cannot be determined solely from a formula, but must be individualized and based on the patient's response and side effects to the medication. For fluphenazine decanoate, the usual dose is 25–50 mg by intramuscular injection every 2–3 weeks. The usual dose for haloperidol decanoate is 100–200 mg intramuscularly every 4 weeks.

POSSIBLE SIDE EFFECTS

Haloperidol decanoate and fluphenazine decanoate are long-acting antipsychotics that exert their action for several weeks. The advantage of the medication's long action may also be a disadvantage to the patient if there are resultant side effects of the medication. Once the decanoate antipsychotic is administered by injection, it cannot be retrieved or easily reversed. Given these considerations, it is important that the patient be treated initially with short-acting haloperidol or fluphenazine before receivIng decanoate injections.

- *Drowsiness and feeling of tiredness.* Generally, high-potency antipsychotics such as haloperidol and fluphenazine do not induce as much drowsiness as the low-potency antipsychotics such as **chlorpromazine** (Thorazine). If excessive drowsiness occurs, the patient's dosage may need to be reduced. Usually, patients develop tolerance to the medication's side effects.

- *Extrapyramidal side effects.* Conventional antipsychotics, especially the high-potency agents such as haloperidol and fluphenazine, can induce abnormal movements that mimic Parkinson's disease. These **Parkinson-like symptoms** include muscle stiffness, rigidity, tremor, drooling, and a masklike face. The Parkinson-like symptoms and other types of involuntary movements are referred to as **extrapyramidal symptoms** (EPS). EPS may be treated, and prevented with *anticholinergic agents* (also called antiparkinson agents), including **benztropine** (Cogentin), **diphenhydramine** (Benadryl), **trihexyphenidyl** (Artane), and **procyclidine** (Kemadrin).

  Dystonia, which occurs shortly after the patient starts an antipsychotic medication, is another form of EPS. It is often manifested by a sudden spasm of the tongue, jaw, and neck. It is not an allergic reaction to the antipsychotic medication. Although a dystonic reaction may be painful and frightening, it can be rapidly reversed with an injection of an anticholinergic medication, such as benztropine or diphenhydramine. With a dystonic reaction, the patient should immediately seek medical attention.

  Akathisia is an inner-driven restlessness caused by antipsychotics. Patients describe it as a feeling of nervousness, with the need to pace and the inability to sit still, and may complain of muscular discomfort. Akathisia can often be misdiagnosed as psychotic agitation. Akathisia responds poorly to anticholinergic medications. Reduction in antipsychotic dose is the usual approach to treating akathisia. **Propranolol** (Inderal), a **beta-blocker,** however, may be helpful for some patients.

- *Gastrointestinal side effects.* Patients may experience dry mouth, nausea, loss of appetite, and constipation. These side effects usually subside over time as the patient develops tolerance to them and may be controlled by reducing the dosage if symptoms persist.

- *Photosensitivity.* Antipsychotics may sensitize the skin (**photosensitivity**) and make it more susceptible to sunburn. Photosensitivity may be more frequent with fluphenazine than with haloperidol. Patients should avoid prolong exposure to the sun and use a sunscreen with a high sun protection factor.

- *Skin rash.* When an allergic skin rash develops, the patient should contact the physician immediately. The physician may prescribe an antihistamine, instructing the patient to take it until the antipsychotic is eliminated from the body.

- *Weight gain.* Antipsychotic medications may induce weight gain in some patients. If weight gain becomes a problem, the patient should discuss it with his or her physician.

- *Other side effects.* Haloperidol and fluphenazine may induce elevated levels of prolactin, a hormone that stimulates breast enlargement and milk secretion. When prolactin levels are elevated, breast enlargement and milk secretion may occur in both women and men. Increased levels of prolactin may also cause sexual dysfunction in men and women and irregular menses in women.

POSSIBLE ADVERSE REACTIONS

- *Tardive dyskinesia (TD).* One of the most worrisome side effects of the conventional antipsychotics is tardive dyskinesia. Although it can occur early on, TD is by definition a late-onset movement disorder produced by antipsychotics. The movements, usually involving the mouth, tongue, or extremities, are involuntary and repetitive. Apparently, a higher incidence of TD is associated with age, women, and cumulative doses and prolonged treatment with antipsychotic medications. With early detection of TD, the patient may be switched to an atypical antipsychotic, such as clozapine, which rarely causes this disorder.

- *Seizures.* Antipsychotics can lower seizure threshold and precipitate seizures in susceptible individuals. High-potency antipsychotics such as haloperidol and fluphenazine are associated with lower incidences of seizures than low-potency antipsychotics such as chlorpromazine. For patients with a history of seizures, the use of antipsychotics must be carefully considered and monitored.

- *Neuroleptic malignant syndrome (NMS).* The symptoms of NMS, a rare, toxic reaction to antipsychotics, are severe muscle stiffness, rigidity, elevated body temperature, increased heart rate and blood pressure, and increased sweating. NMS may lead to delirium and coma. It may be fatal if medical intervention is not immediately provided. Hence, NMS must be recognized early, for it is a medical emergency requiring immediate cessation of the antipsychotic, timely hospitalization, and intensive medical treatment.

- *Heatstroke.* Patients may be more susceptible to heatstroke while taking an antipsychotic. It usually occurs in patients who are exposed to very warm temperatures or become dehydrated. To prevent heatstroke, especially during hot weather, patients should drink plenty of fluids and stay in cooler environments.

PREGNANCY AND BREAST FEEDING

Haloperidol and fluphenazine are classified in **Category C** of the U.S. Food and Drug Administration (FDA) Pregnancy Risk Categories. To date, there are no clinical studies, or there is inadequate information, to determine the extent of risks of haloperidol and fluphenazine with pregnancy. In animal studies, however, some fetal abnormalities were found after maternal exposure to haloperidol and fluphenazine. Interpretation of these animal studies in regard to human risk is unclear. When haloperidol or fluphenazine is prescribed during pregnancy, the long-acting decanoate injections are not recommended because of the risks involved.

Haloperidol and fluphenazine are excreted in breast milk. Therefore, it is recommended that women receiving haloperidol or fluphenazine decanoate injections not breastfeed.

If you have any questions about this handout, please consult your physician.

INFORMATION ABOUT

BUPROPION (WELLBUTRIN, WELLBUTRIN SR, WELLBUTRIN XL)

FOR PATIENTS AND FAMILIES

Bupropion (Wellbutrin) is an effective antidepressant for treatment of many types of depressive disorders, but it also has other clinical uses. It is also used for the treatment of attention-deficit/hyperactivity disorder (ADHD) and, under the trade name **Zyban**, is prescribed for smoking cessation to help smokers with nicotine dependence. Bupropion is not, however, effective in treating panic disorders, anxiety disorders, obsessive-compulsive disorder, and eating disorders.

Bupropion (Wellbutrin) is available in sustained-release (Wellbutrin SR) and extended-release (Wellbutrin XL) tablets. Wellbutrin SR can be administered twice daily, and Wellbutrin XL once a day. Not only are the sustained- and extended-release preparations convenient for dosing, but they may have a lower risk of inducing seizures at higher doses than with immediate-release bupropion.

Bupropion, like other antidepressants, exerts its action in the brain. It is hypothesized that depression may be caused by diminished levels of certain neurotransmitters in the brain. It is unclear exactly how bupropion works. It is thought that bupropion blocks the reuptake of one or more neurotransmitters from going back into brain cells (neurons) and thereby prevents their breakdown. If the patient's depression is due to low levels of a neurotransmitter, increasing the levels of that neurotransmitter may treat the depression. Enhancing the neurotransmitter then facilitates the brain in undergoing changes that ultimately relieve the depression. The lag time for the brain to normalize may explain why antidepressants take weeks before their full effects are seen.

Bupropion is marketed under the brand names Wellbutrin, Wellbutrin SR, and Wellbutrin XL. Bupropion immediate- and sustained-release tablets are available in generic preparations from various manufacturers, but Wellbutrin XL is only available by the brand. Bupropion comes in 75- and 100-mg tablets in the immediate-release form; 100-, 150- and 200-mg tablets in the sustained-release (SR) form, and 150- and 300-mg tablets in the extended-release (XL) form.

HOW BUPROPION IS PRESCRIBED

The usual starting dosage of immediate-release bupropion is 200 mg/day (100 mg twice a day), with the dosage increasing to a target of 300 mg/day (100 mg three times a day) by day four. The initial dose of the SR or XL form is 150 mg once a day in the morning. If the initial dose is adequately tolerated, the dosage is increased to 300 mg/day, given as 150 mg twice a day with Wellbutrin SR or 300 mg once a day with Wellbutrin XL. Any single dose of bupropion should not exceed 150 mg for the immediate-release formulation and 200 mg for the sustained-release tablets. The maximum recommended daily dosage for Wellbutrin is 400 mg/day and for Wellbutrin SR and XL, 450 mg/day. Given the dosing convenience and fewer side effects of the sustained- and extended-release formulations, physicians are mostly prescribing Wellbutrin SR and Wellbutrin XL.

PROPER USE OF YOUR MEDICATION

Storing Your Medication

- Keep your medication in a tamper-resistant vial and out of reach of children.
- Store your medication so as to keep it from excessive heat, moisture, and direct light.
- Keep your medication in its original prescription vial with the label intact to prevent others from taking the medication inadvertently.

Taking Your Medication

- Take your medication as instructed by your physician. Do not abruptly stop taking your medication without telling your physician. Discontinuation of your medication may result in relapse. As with all antidepressants, it may take up to 3 weeks for bupropion to achieve full effect, and improvement may continue for 12 weeks.
- If you missed a dose, take it as soon as possible. However, if it is near the time of your next dose, skip the dose you missed and go back to your regular dosing schedule, but do not double-up the dose. Any single dose of bupropion should not exceed 150 mg for the immediate-release formulation and 200 mg for the sustained-release preparation. Take bupropion sustained-release tablets in two divided doses, separated by 8–12 hours between successive doses. There should be an interval of 24 hours between successive doses with Wellbutrin XL.
- You may take bupropion with or without food. If bupropion upsets your stomach, take it at mealtime. Swallow the sustained-release tablet whole; do not crush or cut it.

Use of Alcohol and Other Medications

Individuals should refrain from alcohol consumption while taking antidepressants. Alcohol is a depressant and may oppose the action of the medication. Excessive alcohol use may also potentiate the risk of seizure with bupropion (see "Possible Adverse Reactions").

Certain medications, including over-the-counter medicines, may interact with the bupropion. The drug interaction may lower the blood level of the affected drug and decrease the drug's effectiveness; or it may elevate the blood level of the affected drug and cause toxicity. When bupropion is combined with certain medications, it may increase or worsen some side effects. Inform your physician of all the prescription and over-the-counter medications you are taking.

Patients taking bupropion should *never* take a **monoamine oxidase inhibitor** (MAOI) antidepressant. The combination may produce severe elevation of blood pressure, fever, and possible seizures. The reaction may be fatal.

It is important to note that bupropion is the same drug used for smoking cessation under the trade name Zyban. Do not use Zyban with Wellbutrin or with any other medication that contains bupropion.

POSSIBLE SIDE EFFECTS

- *Insomnia*. This side effect is apparently the most common complaint. It is easily managed by dosing bupropion in the late afternoon or evening, rather than closer to bedtime. If the insomnia persists, the physician may prescribe a hypnotic agent to improve the patient's sleep. **Trazodone**, a sedating antidepressant, is often prescribed briefly in low doses to help with sleep. Other hypnotic agents that may be used include **diphenhydramine** (Benadryl), a benzodiazepine such as **temazepam** (Restoril), zolpidem (Ambien), or **zaleplon** (Sonata).

- *Restlessness, anxiety, and agitation.* Patients may experience some degree of these side effects, especially shortly after starting therapy. Usually, these side effects are mild and tend to subside over time, but if they persist, the patient should discuss the problem with his or her physician.
- *Sexual dysfunction.* Bupropion usually does not cause sexual dysfunction (i.e., decreased sex drive, delayed ejaculation, or delayed orgasm). As a matter of fact, bupropion is a good alternative for patients who develop sexual dysfunction while taking another antidepressant. Although some patients may be hesitant to discuss their sexual problems, they are encouraged to do so with their doctor.
- *Weight changes and appetite.* Some patients may experience altered appetite or weight loss while taking bupropion. Generally, this side effect is brief, and bupropion is not a good appetite-suppressant for people on a diet.
- *Other side effects* may include headache, tremors, dizziness, dry mouth, and rapid heart rate.

POSSIBLE ADVERSE REACTIONS

- *Seizures.* At higher doses, bupropion is associated with seizures. The incidence of seizures is about 4 per 1,000 patients treated with immediate-release bupropion at dosages below 450 mg/day. The rate, however, increases to 4 per 100 when the dosage is increased above 450 mg/day. The rate of seizures is about 1 per 1,000 patients at a dosage below 400 mg/day for the sustained-release formulation. The risk of seizures is also greater in patients with a history of seizure disorder, bulimia, anorexia, and a history of head trauma. Use of stimulants, alcohol, and cocaine may also predispose the patient to risk of seizures.

  To reduce the risk of seizures, any single dose and the total daily dose of bupropion should not exceed 150 mg and 450 mg for the immediate-release formulation and 200 mg and 400 mg for the sustained-release preparation. It must be administered with caution to patients with a history of seizure, bulimia, or anorexia; patients who are taking medications that may lower the seizure threshold; and patients with a history of drug use.

- *Activation of mania or hypomania.* Antidepressants in general can trigger a manic or hypomanic (less severe form of mania) episode in patients who are in the depressed phase of a bipolar illness. However, bupropion is associated with a much lower risk of triggering mania or hypomania than, for example, tricyclic antidepressants. Nevertheless, patients with bipolar disorder who are taking bupropion should be aware of this potential reaction.

PREGNANCY AND BREAST FEEDING

Bupropion is in **Category B** of the FDA Pregnancy Risk Categories. There are no clinical studies, and there is inadequate information, on the use of bupropion in women, and so risk during pregnancy cannot be determined. Findings from animal studies of bupropion are negative for fetal abnormalities. Bupropion, however, should be used during pregnancy only if the benefits outweigh the risk.

Bupropion is excreted in breast milk. Women taking bupropion should not breastfeed. The long-term effects of bupropion to the developing infant are unknown.

If you have any questions about this handout, please consult your physician.

INFORMATION ABOUT

CLOMIPRAMINE (ANAFRANIL)

FOR PATIENTS AND FAMILIES

Clomipramine (Anafranil) is one of many antidepressants in the family of tricyclic antidepressants (**tricyclic** refers to their three-ring chemical structure). Clomipramine is primarily used in treating obsessive-compulsive disorder (OCD). Interestingly, the U.S. Drug and Food Administration (FDA) approved clomipramine only for the treatment of OCD, and not depression, although physicians prescribe it for depression. It has been proven effective for treating depression. It is also used to treat agoraphobia (abnormal fear of being in open or public places from which escape might be difficult or embarrassing), panic disorder, and other types of depressive disorders.

It has been hypothesized that the symptoms of OCD may be related to serotonin, a neurotransmitter, in the brain. It is unclear what exact role serotonin plays in OCD, but changes in serotonin levels in the brain effected by medicines like clomipramine are important in mediating treatment-response in OCD. Clomipramine has been the standard in treatment of OCD for over two decades.

Clomipramine is available in generic preparations from different manufacturers, but it is marketed under the brand name of **Anafranil**. It is available in 25-, 50-, and 75-mg capsules.

HOW CLOMIPRAMINE IS PRESCRIBED

The usual starting dose for treating OCD is 25–50 mg administered in a single dose at bedtime. The dose is gradually increased during the first 2 weeks in increments of 25 mg/day, depending on clinical response and tolerability to side effects, to about 100 mg/day administered in divided doses. At higher dosages, clomipramine is best taken in two or three divided doses at mealtime to minimize gastrointestinal side effects. The maximum dosage for clomipramine should not exceed 250 mg/day.

PROPER USE OF YOUR MEDICATION

Storing Your Medication

- Keep your medication in a tamper-resistant vial and out of reach of children. Overdosage of clomipramine, a tricyclic antidepressant, is extremely dangerous, especially in infants and young children.
- Store your medication from excessive heat, moisture, and direct light.
- Keep your medication in its original prescription vial with the label intact to prevent others from taking the medication inadvertently.

Taking Your Medication

- Take your medication as instructed by your physician. Do not abruptly stop taking your medication without telling your physician. Discontinuation of your medication may result in relapse. Abrupt discontinuation of clomipramine may cause unpleasant symptoms. Although not indicative of addiction, the dosage may need to be decreased gradually before discontinuation of clomipramine.

- It may take 4–6 weeks of treatment before the therapeutic benefits of clomipramine are seen, and maximum therapeutic benefits are generally obtained in 8–16 weeks.
- If you miss a dose, take it as soon as possible. However, if it is close to your next dose, skip it and go back to your regular dosing schedule, but do not double-up the dose.
- Clomipramine may be taken with or without food. If it upsets your stomach, take it at mealtime.

Use of Alcohol and Other Medications

Individuals should refrain from alcohol consumption while taking antidepressants. Alcohol is a depressant and may oppose the action of the medication.

Certain medications, including over-the-counter medicines, may adversely interact with clomipramine. The drug interaction may *lower* the blood level of the affected drug and decrease its effectiveness; or, it may *elevate* the blood level of the affected drug and cause toxicity. There are some drugs that when combined with clomipramine may exacerbate some side effects. Inform your doctor of all the prescription and over-the-counter medications you are taking. If you have questions about your medications, consult your physician or pharmacist.

POSSIBLE SIDE EFFECTS

- *Drowsiness and sedation.* Patients taking clomipramine frequently report side effects of drowsiness and sedation. For this reason, the medication is initiated at a low dose and administered at bedtime to minimize daytime sedation. As the dosage is increased, clomipramine is administered in divided doses. A larger portion of the divided dose may be taken at bedtime to reduce daytime sedation.
- *Anticholinergic side effects.* When clomipramine interferes with the part of the nervous system—the cholinergic system—that regulates those particular body functions, it produces unwanted side effects. Drugs that inhibit the function of the cholinergic nervous system produce **anticholinergic side effects.** These side effects include dry mouth, blurred vision, disturbance of **accommodation** (failure of the eye to adjust when looking at nearby objects), constipation, urinary retention and hesitation, and palpitations. Furthermore, excessive anticholinergic action may produce confusion, especially in elderly patients.
- *Gastrointestinal (GI) side effects.* Nausea, dry mouth, loss of appetite, constipation, and heartburn are common GI complaints from taking clomipramine. As discussed above, dry mouth and constipation are anticholinergic side effects of the medication. Taking clomipramine at mealtime may reduce nausea. Using a bulk laxative, such as Metamucil, or a stool softener, increasing exercise, and drinking adequate liquid may prevent constipation.
- *Weight changes.* Weight gain was reported in 18% of patients receiving clomipramine. If weight gain is problematic, and a program of reducing caloric intake and increasing exercise does not control the weight, the physician may switch the patient to another antidepressant without this side effect.
- *Orthostatic hypotension.* Low blood pressure due to a postural change is known as **orthostatic hypotension**. Clomipramine may oppose the action of the body to elevate blood pressure when there is a change in position. When blood pressure cannot be elevated rapidly to compensate for a postural change as the patient rises from bed or stands up, orthostatic hypotension results. A drop in blood pressure can cause the individual to feel light-headed and dizzy, and sometimes faint and fall. By learning to rise slowly to allow the blood pressure to adjust, the patient can avoid or minimize orthostatic hypotension. Orthostatic hypotension from clomipramine is usually mild. Elderly patients and those taking larger doses may be more susceptible to this side effect.
- *Sexual dysfunction.* Clomipramine may cause sexual dysfunction, including impotence, delayed ejaculation, diminished libido, and anorgasmia (inability to achieve orgasm). Although some patients may be hesitant to discuss their sexual problems, they are encouraged to so with their doctor. The physician may suggest switching to another antidepressant with a lower incidence of sexual problems.

> **Warning**:   Clomipramine may cause drowsiness and dizziness. Patients must exercise caution when engaging in daily activities that require mental alertness, such as operating a motor vehicle. It is recommended that the patients do not engage in hazardous tasks until they are reasonably certain that their medication does not adversely affect their performance or impair their judgment.

POSSIBLE ADVERSE REACTIONS

- *Seizures.* Clomipramine, as with other tricyclic antidepressants, may lower the seizure threshold and increase the risk of seizures in susceptible individuals. The risk may be further enhanced when clomipramine is combined with other medicines that also lower seizure threshold. Albeit seizures are rare with clomipramine, patients with a history of seizure disorder should be monitored closely during treatment.
- *Mania and hypomania.* In patients diagnosed with bipolar disorder, taking clomipramine may precipitate mania or hypomania (less severe form of mania). Although the incidence of triggering mania or hypomania is very low, individuals with a history of bipolar illness should be aware of this adverse reaction while taking clomipramine.
- *Drug interactions.* Patients taking clomipramine should *never* take **monoamine oxidase inhibitor** (MAOI) antidepressants, such as **phenelzine** (Nardil), **tranylcypromine** (Parnate), and **isocarboxazid** (Marplan). This combination may result in severe elevation of blood pressure, fever, and possible seizures. If medical intervention and discontinuation the medications are not immediate, the reaction may be fatal. Clomipramine must be used cautiously in combination with selective serotonin reuptake inhibitor (SSRI) antidepressants, such as **fluoxetine** (Prozac) and **paroxetine** (Paxil). The combination may precipitate an adverse reaction known as **serotonin syndrome,** with symptoms that include confusion, restlessness, tremors, sweating, diarrhea, and fever.

PREGNANCY AND BREAST FEEDING

Clomipramine is classified in **Category C** of the U.S. Food and Drug Administration (FDA) Pregnancy Risk Categories. It is given this classification because there are no clinical studies in women, nor is there adequate information, to determine the risk of clomipramine during pregnancy. Animal studies have found some abnormalities in the fetus of animals during maternal exposure to clomipramine. Interpretation of the animal studies to human risks, however, is unclear. Therefore, clomipramine should be prescribed during pregnancy only if the benefits outweigh the potential risks.

Clomipramine is excreted in breastmilk. It is recommended that women who breastfeed not take clomipramine.

If you have any questions about this handout, please consult your physician.

Information About

Mirtazapine (Remeron)

for Patients and Families

Mirtazapine (Remeron) is an antidepressant for treatment of many types of depressive disorders. It is also effective in treating anxiety disorders, including panic disorder. Patients with depression and anxiety usually respond well to mirtazapine. It has been suggested that mirtazapine's onset of action may be more rapid than that of other antidepressants, including selective serotonin reuptake inhibitors (SSRIs), such as fluoxetine (Prozac). Furthermore, mirtazapine's action may complement the action of other antidepressants, so that it may be used to augment the antidepressant effect of another antidepressant.

It is hypothesized that diminished levels of one or more neurotransmitters in the brain may be the cause of depression. Mirtazapine's antidepressant effect may be related to its action in increasing the levels of neurotransmitters. As more neurotransmitters are made available, the brain undergoes changes that ultimately relieve depression. The lag time for the brain to normalize explains why antidepressants, including mirtazapine, may take weeks before their full effects are achieved.

Mirtazapine is available in tablet form as the brand **Remeron,** and generically as well, in strengths of 15, 30, and 45 mg. It is also available in rapidly dissolving tablets (**Remeron Sol Tab**) in the same strengths. Remeron Sol Tabs dissolve in the mouth and eliminate the need to swallow a pill.

HOW MIRTAZAPINE IS PRESCRIBED

The recommended starting dose of mirtazapine is 15 mg administered in a single dose, preferably prior to bedtime. Some physicians may use a higher starting dosage of 30 mg/day because there appears to be less sedation at the higher dose. This paradox may be due to the difference in mirtazapine's activity at lower doses than at higher doses. If response is not achieved after 1–2 weeks, the dosage may be increased by 15 mg/day until a maximum dosage of 45 mg/day is reached.

PROPER USE OF YOUR MEDICATION

Storing Your Medication
- Keep your medication in a tamper-resistant vial and out of reach of children.
- Store your medication so as to keep it from excessive heat, moisture, and direct light.
- Keep your medication in its original prescription vial with the label intact to prevent others from taking the medication inadvertently.

Taking Your Medication
- Take your medication as instructed by your physician. Do not abruptly stop taking your medication without telling your physician. Discontinuation of your medication may result in relapse. Mirtazapine, like all antidepressants, may take several weeks to achieve its full effect.

- If you miss a dose, take it as soon as possible. However, if it is close to your next dose, skip it and go back to your regular dosing schedule, but do not double-up the dose.
- Your antidepressant may be taken with or without food. If it upsets your stomach, take it at mealtime.

Use of Alcohol and Other Medications

Individuals should refrain from using alcohol while taking antidepressants. Alcohol is a depressant and may oppose the intended action of the antidepressant medication.

Certain medications, including over-the-counter medicines, may interact with mirtazapine. The drug interaction may *lower* the blood level of the affected drug and decrease the drug's effectiveness; or, it may *elevate* the blood level of the affected drug and cause toxicity. When certain drugs are combined with mirtazapine, they may make some side effects worse. Inform your physician of all the prescription and over-the-counter medications you are taking.

Patients taking mirtazapine should *never* take a type of antidepressants known as **monoamine oxidase inhibitors** (MAOIs), such as **phenelzine** (Nardil), **tranylcypromine** (Parnate), and **isocarboxazid** (Marplan). The combination of mirtazapine and MAOI may produce a severe reaction, resulting in high blood pressure, fever, and possible seizures.

POSSIBLE SIDE EFFECTS

- *Drowsiness and sedation.* Drowsiness and sedation are common side effects from mirtazapine. For this reason, the medication is best taken at bedtime to minimize daytime sedation.
- *Gastrointestinal side effects.* Dry mouth is a frequent complaint, but constipation appears to be less frequent.
- *Increased appetite and weight gain.* In the first 6 weeks, mirtazapine may enhance appetite for some patients, which may result in weight gain. For patients whose depressive symptoms include poor appetite and weight loss, this effect may be beneficial. For others, weight gain may be problematic. If a strategy of decreasing caloric intake and increasing exercise does not control the weight, the physician may switch the patient to another antidepressant that is weight-neutral.
- *Increased cholesterol and triglycerides.* In clinical trials, about 15% of patients treated with mirtazapine had significant increase in their cholesterol, and about 6% of patients experienced an increase in triglycerides. It may be necessary to switch the patient to another antidepressant if levels of cholesterol and triglycerides are significantly elevated. If discontinuing mirtazapine is not a viable option, the patient may benefit from a lipid-lowering agent like atorvastatin (Lipitor) to reduce the cardiovascular risks of elevated levels of cholesterol and triglycerides.
- *Orthostatic hypotension.* Low blood pressure due to a postural change is known as **orthostatic hypotension**. Mirtazapine may oppose the body's ability to elevate blood pressure when there is a change in position. If the blood pressure cannot elevate in time to compensate for the change in position as the individual rises from a lying or sitting position, orthostatic hypotension ensues. As a result, the individual feels light-headed and dizzy, has a rapid heart rate, and may faint and fall. By learning to rise slowly to allow the blood pressure to adjust, the patient may avoid or minimize orthostatic hypotension. Mirtazapine-induced orthostatic hypotension is usually mild, but elderly patients and patients who are taking larger doses may be more susceptible to this side effect.
- *Dizziness.* Up to 7% of patients taking mirtazapine report symptoms of dizziness. In some of these cases, the dizziness may be caused by orthostatic hypotension.
- *Elevation of liver enzymes.* In clinical trials, approximately 2% of patients taking mirtazapine were found to have elevation of a particular liver enzyme (alanine transaminase, or ALT). Elevation of liver enzymes is generally indicative of compromised liver function. The majority of these patients did not develop any liver problems when mirtazapine was discontinued, and in other cases the enzyme levels returned to normal despite continued treatment.

Warning: Mirtazapine may cause drowsiness and dizziness. Patients must exercise caution when engaging in daily activities that require mental alertness, such as operating a motor vehicle. It is recommended that patients do not engage in hazardous tasks until they are reasonably certain that their medication does not adversely affect their performance or impair their judgment.

POSSIBLE ADVERSE REACTIONS

- *Seizures.* Mirtazapine, like other antidepressants, may lower the seizure threshold and increase the risk of seizures in susceptible individuals. The risk may be further enhanced when mirtazapine is combined with other medicines that may also lower the seizure threshold. Patients with a history of seizure disorder should be monitored closely while taking mirtazapine, albeit seizures are rare.
- *Agranulocytosis.* Granulocytes, a type of white blood cell in the body's immune system, are important for fighting infections. When these cells are significantly decreased (**agranulocytosis**), the immune system is compromised and the individual may be susceptible to life-threatening infections.

  During clinical trials, two patients treated with mirtazapine developed agranulocytosis with signs and symptoms of infections. A third patient developed low granulocytes without signs of infection. In all three cases, there were no serious consequences when the antidepressant was discontinued. Although mirtazapine-induced agranulocytosis is extremely rare, the patient should notify the physician if he or she develops a persistent sore throat, fever, or other lingering signs of infection while taking mirtazapine.
- *Mania and hypomania.* In patients with bipolar disorder, when treating the depressive phase of the illness with antidepressants, there is a risk that the medication may precipitate mania or hypomania (less severe form of mania). Although the incidence of triggering mania or hypomania is rare during treatment with mirtazapine, individuals with a history of bipolar illness should be aware of this potential reaction.

PREGNANCY AND BREAST FEEDING

Mirtazapine is in **Category C** of the U.S. Food and Drug Administration (FDA) Pregnancy Risk Categories. It is given this classification because there are no clinical studies in women, nor is there adequate information, to determine the risk of this drug during pregnancy. Animal studies have found some abnormalities in the fetus during maternal exposure to mirtazapine. However, interpretation of animal studies in regard to human risks is unclear. The risk of mirtazapine to the fetus cannot be ruled out, and the antidepressant should be prescribed during pregnancy only if the benefits outweigh the potential risk.

It is not known if mirtazapine is excreted in breast milk. Women taking mirtazapine should not breastfeed.

If you have any questions about this handout, please consult your physician.

INFORMATION ABOUT

MONOAMINE OXIDASE INHIBITORS (MAOIs)

FOR PATIENTS AND FAMILIES

○ **Isocarboxazid (Marplan)**   ○ **Phenelzine (Nardil)**

○ **Tranylcypromine (Parnate)**   ○ **Selegiline (Eldepryl)**

Monoamine oxidase inhibitors (MAOIs) represent an older class of antidepressants that have essentially been replaced by safer agents for treatment of depression. Physicians generally do not initiate MAOIs as first-line antidepressants because of their serious side effects, involving potentially dangerous interactions with certain foods and medications.

MAOIs are indicated for treatment of severe forms of depression, such as **atypical depression**, that have not responded to other antidepressants. In atypical depression, the patient is overly sensitive to rejection, has difficulty with expressing emotions, is prone to labile or fragile moods, oversleeps and overeats, feels extreme fatigue or "leaden paralysis," and is highly emotional and reactive to daily events. When patients with atypical depression do not respond to a selective serotonin reuptake inhibitor (SSRI) antidepressant, such as fluoxetine (Prozac), an MAOI may be indicated and often may be effective. MAOIs may also be efficacious, when other antidepressants have not been effective, in treating anxiety and panic attacks, agoraphobia, and eating disorders such as bulimia.

Monoamine oxidases are enzymes distributed throughout the body, including the brain. These enzymes are responsible for breaking down specific chemicals in the body, including two important neurotransmitters in the brain: **norepinephrine** and **serotonin**. Norepinephrine and serotonin are just a few of many neurotransmitters in the central nervous system. Decreased concentrations of neurotransmitters in the brain may be associated with depression and the aforementioned disorders. *Monoamine oxidase inhibitors,* as the term implies, work by inhibiting, or "blocking," this enzyme system, thus increasing the levels of neurotransmitters, including norepinephrine and serotonin. As more neurotransmitters are made available, the brain undergoes changes that ultimately relieve depression. The lag time for the brain to normalize may explain why antidepressants, including MAOIs, may take weeks before achieving their full effects.

Three MAOIs—**phenelzine** (Nardil), **tranylcypromine** (Parnate), and **isocarboxazid** (Marplan)—are approved by the U.S. Food and Drug Administration (FDA) for treatment of depression. Another MAOI—**selegiline** (Eldepryl)—is approved for treatment of **Parkinson's disease** (a neurologic disorder that affects movement). When selegiline is used for treatment of depression, higher doses than those used for treatment of Parkinson's disease are necessary.

Phenelzine, tranylcypromine, and isocarboxazid are available only under their brands. Selegiline is available under the trade names **Eldepryl** and **Carbex,** as well as from different generic manufacturers. MAOIs are available only in the following strengths: phenelzine, 15 mg; tranylcypromine and isocarboxazid, 10 mg; and selegiline, 5 mg.

HOW MAOIs ARE PRESCRIBED

MAOIs should not be taken concomitantly with other antidepressants. The combination is hazardous and may precipitate a severe reaction. MAOIs should not be taken within 14 days after stopping another antidepressant, which allows sufficient time for it to be eliminated from the body. Also, at least 2 weeks must be allowed after stopping an MAOI before another antidepressant may be started.

The dosages for MAOIs are carefully individualized to the patient's clinical response and tolerability to the medication. Physicians usually start slowly with low doses and increase the dose gradually to allow patients to adapt to the side effects. It may take several weeks before the patient feels a significant response. The dosage ranges for MAOIs are as follows: phenelzine, 45 to 90 mg/day; tranylcypromine, 30 to 60 mg/day; isocarboxazid, 40–60 mg/ day; and selegiline, 20–50 mg/day. The total daily doses are usually administered in two or three divided doses.

PROPER USE OF YOUR MEDICATION

Storing Your Medication

- Keep your medication in a tamper-resistant vial and out of reach of children.
- Store your medication so as to keep it from excessive heat, moisture, and direct light.
- Keep your medication in its original prescription vial with the label intact to prevent others from taking the medication inadvertently.

Taking Your Medication

- Take your medication exactly as instructed by your physician. Do not abruptly stop taking your medication without consulting your physician. Abrupt discontinuation of your medication may result in unpleasant withdrawal symptoms and relapse of symptoms. MAOI antidepressants need to be decreased gradually before stopping the medication.
- An MAOI antidepressant, like all antidepressants, may take several weeks to achieve full effect.
- If you missed a dose, take it as soon as possible. However, if it is near the time of your next dose, skip the dose you missed and go back to your regular dosing schedule, but do not double-up the dose.
- Your antidepressant may be taken with food or without food. If it upsets your stomach, take it at mealtime.

Avoid Tyramine-Containing Foods

Certain foods and beverages are rich in **tyramine.** Tyramine is a naturally occurring substance generally derived from the aging process of food and alcohol. Tyramine is broken down in the intestines by monoamine oxidase enzymes before any significant amount is absorbed and distributed in the body. However, when an MAOI is present, the enzyme system is blocked throughout the body, including in the patient's intestines. As foods high in tyramine are consumed, large amounts of tyramine are absorbed and distributed unchecked. High levels of tyramine can cause blood vessels to constrict, thus elevating blood pressure. When blood pressure becomes dangerously elevated and goes untreated, a **hypertensive crisis** ensues. Patients taking MAOI antidepressants minimize the risks of a hypertensive reaction by avoiding certain foods and beverages high in tyramine (see Table 1).

Table 1. Dietary Restrictions When Taking Monoamine Oxidase Inhibitors (MAOIs)

Tyramine-Containing Foods That Must Be Avoided

- Cheese and cheese-containing foods (present in Italian dishes, salad dressings, and sauces) *Cream cheese, cottage cheese, and ricotta are safe.*
- Beer (including some nonalcoholic), ale, red wine (especially Chianti), sherry, cognac, and Vermouth
- Aged meats (e.g., corned beef), processed meats, and nonfresh meats
- Sausages, including salami, pepperoni, bologna, and summer sausages
- Fermented or aged fish (e.g., pickled herring)
- Beef liver or chicken liver, including liverwurst
- Fava or broad bean pods
- Meat extracts or yeast extracts (e.g., Marmite) *Yeasts in baked goods are safe.*
- Tofu, fermented bean curd (in miso soup and soybean curd), and shrimp paste
- Sauerkraut

Foods That Should Be Consumed in Moderation

- Caffeine-containing beverages, including coffee, cola, and tea
- Chocolate
- Yogurt
- Sour cream
- Soy sauce
- Distilled spirits, including vodka, gin, and whiskey
- Smoked fish, including salmon and whitefish
- Ripe avocados and bananas
- Dried fruits, including figs and raisins

Use of Alcohol and Other Medications

Patients taking MAOIs should not drink alcohol. Beer and red wine must definitely be avoided because the combination may cause a sudden rise in blood pressure and a hypertensive crisis.

Certain medications, including over-the-counter medicines, may interact with MAOI antidepressants and must be avoided (see Table 2). The drug interaction can precipitate a potentially fatal hypertensive crisis. Before taking any medications, including over-the-counter medicines and herbal supplements, the patient should always consult with his or her physician or pharmacist. The patient should be sure to inform other physicians that he or she is taking an MAOI.

Table 2. Drug Restrictions When Taking Monoamine Oxidase Inhibitors (MAOIs)

Drugs That Must Be Avoided

- Other antidepressants (e.g., Prozac, Elavil, Effexor, Remeron)
- Meperidine (e.g., Demerol)
- Levodopa (e.g., Sinemet) for Parkinson's disease
- L-Tryptophan (an over-the-counter amino acid promoted for insomnia)
- Methylphenidate (e.g., Ritalin)
- Decongestants in cold/sinus and allergy/hay fever medications
- Bronchodilator inhalants for breathing (e.g., Alupent, Ventolin)
- Epinephrine in local anesthetics, emergency bee-sting kits, injections for treatment of acute asthma (Sus-phrine), and nasal inhalers and solution for nebulizers
- Amphetamines (e.g., Dexedrine)
- Diet pills
- Cocaine

Note. The table lists the common drugs that must be avoided with MAOIs. There may be other medications not listed that can interact with MAOIs. Always consult your physician or pharmacist before taking any medication with an MAOI.

POSSIBLE SIDE EFFECTS

The patient may experience some bothersome side effects from the MAOI antidepressant, especially shortly after beginning therapy, but should not become unduly alarmed. These common side effects usually subside as the individual becomes adjusted to the medication. If the side effect is intolerable or persists, the patient should consult with the physician to reduce the dosage. The patient, however, should understand and recognize the signs and symptoms of more serious reactions (discussed later under "Possible Adverse Reactions") with MAOIs.

- *Orthostatic hypotension.* Low blood pressure due to a postural change is known as **orthostatic hypotension**. MAOIs may oppose the body's ability to raise blood pressure when there is a change in position. If the blood pressure cannot elevate in time to compensate for the change in position as the individual rises from a lying or sitting position, **orthostatic hypotension** ensues. As a result, the individual feels light-headed and dizzy, has a rapid heart rate, and may faint and fall. By learning to rise slowly to allow the blood pressure to adjust, the patient may avoid or minimize orthostatic hypotension. Elderly patients and patients taking larger doses may be more susceptible to this side effect.
- *Insomnia and daytime sleepiness.* For some people, MAOIs may cause sleeping difficulties. Insomnia may be minimized by taking a larger portion of the divided doses in the morning. Other patients, paradoxically, may experience daytime sleepiness. When daytime sleepiness becomes a problem, the larger dose may be taken at night.
- *Gastrointestinal side effects.* Constipation, nausea, dry mouth, diarrhea, heartburn, and abdominal pain can occur.
- *Sexual dysfunction.* MAOIs may induce sexual dysfunction, including impotence, delayed ejaculation, diminished libido, and anorgasmia (inability to achieve orgasm). Although many patients may be hesitant to discuss their sexual problems, they are encouraged to express their concerns to their doctor. The physician may suggest switching to another antidepressant with lower incidences of inducing sexual dysfunction.
- *Withdrawal symptoms.* Abrupt withdrawal of MAOIs may be associated with nausea, vomiting, and flu-like symptoms. These symptoms may be prevented by gradually decreasing the dose before discontinuation.

- *Other possible side effects*: Dizziness, headaches, tremors, muscle twitching, confusion, nervousness, weight gain, urinary retention, and urinary hesitancy can occur. If any of the side effects persist or are intolerable, discuss the symptoms with your physician.

> **Warning**:   MAOIs may cause drowsiness and dizziness. Patients must exercise caution when engaging in activities that require mental alertness, such as operating a motor vehicle. It is recommended that patients do not engage in hazardous tasks until they are reasonably certain that their medication does not adversely affect their performance or impair their judgment.

POSSIBLE ADVERSE REACTIONS

- *Hypertensive crisis.* The major—and the most worrisome—adverse reaction with MAOIs is sudden and dramatic elevation of blood pressure. High blood pressure, or **hypertension,** usually occurs several hours after ingestion of a contraindicated food or medication. Dangerously high blood pressure may cause strokes and other serious cardiovascular sequelae. This kind of malignant high blood pressure is known as a **hypertensive crisis.**

  Patients should learn to recognize the signs and symptoms of high blood pressure. Patients should also learn to take their blood pressure and monitor it on a regular basis. A severe headache is usually the first sign of high blood pressure. Early signs of a hypertensive crisis may include rapid heartbeat (palpitations), sweating, nausea, vomiting, fever, cold and clammy skin, and dilated pupils. When these symptoms occur, discontinue all medications immediately and contact your physician and seek immediate medical attention.

- *Serotonin syndrome.* When two or more drugs that increase serotonin levels are taken together, excessive stimulation of the serotonergic system in the brain may result in a reaction called **serotonin syndrome**. Drugs that increase serotonin include MAOIs; L-tryptophan; amphetamines; SSRIs, such as fluoxetine (Prozac); tricyclic antidepressants, such as amitriptyline (Elavil); and even over-the-counter herbal supplements such as St. John's wort. The combination of an MAOI and an SSRI is especially hazardous and should be avoided. Symptoms of serotonin syndrome include restlessness, confusion, tremors, muscle jerks, and loss of coordination. If the medications are not stopped immediately, the complications of serotonin syndrome may include high fever, muscle rigidity, clotting disorders, and loss of consciousness. In a severe case that goes untreated, the syndrome can be fatal. Patients taking MAOIs should never self-medicate without first consulting with their physician or pharmacist.

PREGNANCY AND BREAST FEEDING

The MAOIs are in **Category C** of the U.S. Food and Drug Administration (FDA) Pregnancy Risk Categories. The MAOIs are given this classification because there are no clinical studies, or there is inadequate information, on MAOI use in women to determine the risk during pregnancy. Animal studies have found some abnormalities in the fetus during maternal exposure to MAOIs. However, interpretation of animal studies in regard to human risks is unclear. The risk of these agents to the fetus cannot be ruled out, and MAOIs should be prescribed during pregnancy only if the benefits outweigh the potential risk.

Tranylcypromine is excreted in breastmilk, but it is not known if the other MAOIs are. Women taking MAOIs should not breastfeed.

If you have any questions about this handout, please consult your physician.

INFORMATION ABOUT

NEFAZODONE (SERZONE) AND TRAZODONE (DESYREL)

FOR PATIENTS AND FAMILIES

Nefazodone (Serzone) and **trazodone** (Desyrel) are antidepressants used in the treatment of major depression. The two antidepressants are similar in the way they work. However, they have different clinical uses. Nefazodone is an effective antidepressant for treating depression complicated by anxiety and sleep disturbance, generalized anxiety disorder, posttraumatic stress disorder, panic disorder, and social phobia. Trazodone, once a widely used antidepressant, has essentially been supplanted by nefazodone for treating depression. The reason is that trazodone is very sedating, and patients have difficulty tolerating the medication. Today, trazodone is mostly used for sleep difficulties. It is effective for treating insomnia induced by the **selective serotonin reuptake inhibitor** (SSRI) antidepressants, such as **fluoxetine** (Prozac) and **sertraline** (Zoloft). Prescribed in low doses, trazodone may benefit sleep and augment the antidepressant effect of the SSRI.

Nefazodone was sold under the brand Serzone, but the manufacturer recently pulled the drug off the market. However, nefazodone is available in generic equivalents from various manufacturers.[1] It comes in 50-, 100-, 150-, 200-, and 300-mg tablets. Trazodone is usually dispensed in the generic form and seldom by the brand, Desyrel. It comes in 50-, 100-, 150-, and 300-mg tablets.

HOW NEFAZODONE AND TRAZODONE ARE PRESCRIBED

The usual starting dose of nefazodone for adults is 100 mg two times daily (200 mg/day). For elderly or debilitated patients, the starting dose is 50 mg two times daily. The dose may be increased at weekly intervals as needed, depending on clinical response. Dosages range from 300 to 600 mg/day.

Trazodone is effective for treating sleep disturbances caused by SSRI antidepressants. For treating insomnia, 50–100 mg of trazodone at bedtime is an effective hypnotic dose.

PROPER USE OF YOUR MEDICATION

Storing Your Medication

- Keep your medication in a tamper-resistant vial and out of reach of children.
- Store your medication so as to keep it from excessive heat, moisture, and direct light.
- Keep your medication in its original prescription vial with the label intact to prevent others from taking the medication inadvertently.

Taking Your Medication

- Take your medication as instructed by your physician. Do not abruptly stop taking your medication without telling your physician. Discontinuation of your medication may result in relapse. It may take up to 2 weeks for the antidepressant to achieve full effect, and improvement may continue for 12 weeks.

---

[1]A watchdog group, Public Citizens, is suing the FDA to take all versions of nefazodone off the market because of the drug's associated risk of liver failure.

Do not abruptly discontinue the antidepressant without consulting with your physician. The dosage of the antidepressant is usually decreased gradually before the medication is stopped completely.

- If you miss a dose, take it as soon as possible. However, if it is near the time of your next dose, skip the dose you missed and go back to your regular dosing schedule, but do not double-up the dose.
- Your antidepressant may be taken with or without food. If it upsets your stomach, take it at mealtime.

Use of Alcohol and Other Medications

Individuals should refrain from using alcohol while taking antidepressants. These medications may produce drowsiness and dizziness. Use of alcohol may make these side effects worse. Furthermore, alcohol is a depressant, and excessive use may oppose the action of the antidepressant.

Certain medications, including over-the-counter medicines, may interact with nefazodone or trazodone. The drug interaction may lower the blood level of the affected drug and decrease the drug's effectiveness; or, it may elevate the blood level of the affected drug and cause toxicity. When certain drugs are combined with nefazodone or trazodone, they may exacerbate some side effects. Inform your physician of all the prescription and over-the-counter medications you are taking. Before self-medicating with an over-the-counter medication, ask your pharmacist if it may be taken concomitantly with your antidepressant.

Patients taking nefazodone or trazodone should not take **monoamine oxidase inhibitor** (MAOI) antidepressants. The combination may produce a severe reaction that may result in elevated blood pressure, fever, and possible seizures.

POSSIBLE SIDE EFFECTS

- *Sedation.* This side effect is a common complaint with trazodone and nefazodone. Trazodone, however, is more sedating than nefazodone. Daytime sedation from nefazodone may be managed by taking a larger portion of the divided dose at bedtime than during the day. Usually, patients adjust to the drowsiness of the antidepressant when it is taken in lower doses and the dose is gradually increased. The patient must observe caution while driving or performing tasks that require alertness.
- *Gastrointestinal side effects.* Nausea, stomach upset, constipation, and dry mouth are frequent side effects of nefazodone and trazodone, but generally these side effects are mild. Gastrointestinal upset may be reduced when these medications are taken with food.
- *Sexual dysfunction.* Nefazodone and trazodone usually do not cause sexual dysfunctions (i.e., decreased sex drive, delayed ejaculation, delayed orgasm). On the contrary, nefazodone is a good alternative for patients who develop sexual dysfunction from other types of antidepressants. If sexual dysfunction occurs, although some patients may be hesitant to discuss their sexual problems, they are encouraged to talk to their physician.
- *Restlessness and jitteriness.* Occasionally, a patient may complain of restlessness and jitteriness while taking nefazodone or trazodone. This side effect may be more common when the patient is taking nefazodone or trazodone and another antidepressant, especially fluoxetine (Prozac).
- *Visual disturbance.* Visual side effects may occur when patients are taking nefazodone. Patients report seeing an afterimage during tracking of moving objects. These visual side effects subside over time. The patient should discuss this with his or her physician if it is intolerable.

POSSIBLE ADVERSE REACTIONS

- *Liver failure.* Cases of life-threatening liver failure resulting in deaths and liver transplant have been reported in patients taking nefazodone. These cases have prompted the FDA to require all manufacturers to put a "black box" warning on nefazodone labeling. The new warning states that patients taking nefazodone have a higher risk of developing liver failure than those untreated: the rate of liver failure in those treated is about three to four times greater than in those untreated. The link between liver failure and nefazodone is unclear, but it may be related to a hypersensitivity to the medication. Patients who have active liver disease or elevated liver enzymes should not take nefazodone. Patients whose liver function is currently normal but who have a history of liver disease should have their liver function closely monitored while taking nefazodone. While taking nefazodone, patients should be alert to the signs and symptoms of liver dysfunction and report their physicians immediately. Symptoms may include yellowing of the skin and whites of the eyes (jaundice), tiredness, poor appetite, flulike symptoms, nausea, abdominal pain, and abnormally dark urine.

- *Priapism.* Some medications can cause a rare condition in males that results in a prolonged, uncontrollable, painful penile erection. Trazodone may induce priapism, and the incidence of priapism associated with trazodone is about 1 per 6,000 patients. Although there has not been a report of nefazodone-induced priapism, this effect is still of concern because nefazodone is structurally similar to trazodone. Male patients taking trazodone or nefazodone who experience an uncontrolled erection persisting over 1 hour should seek immediate medical attention. If not treated promptly, priapism may result in permanent impotence due to damage of vascular structures in the penis.

- *Serious drug interactions.* Taking nefazodone with some medications concomitantly may increase the serum levels of these agents because nefazodone inhibits their metabolism. The blood levels of **astemizole** (Hismanal), **ketoconazole** (Nizoral), **cisapride** (Propulsid), and **pimozide** (Orap) may be elevated significantly by nefazodone, and toxicity may occur. There is a potential risk of cardiac arrhythmias from the elevated levels of these drugs. In addition, nefazodone may significantly elevate the levels of **alprazolam** (Xanax) and **triazolam** (Halcion). If any of these medications are prescribed with nefazodone, the patient should consult with the physician before taking them.

PREGNANCY AND BREAST FEEDING

Nefazodone and trazodone are classified in **Category C** of the U.S. Food and Drug Administration (FDA) Pregnancy Risk Categories. They are given this classification because there are no clinical studies in women, nor is there adequate information, on use of nefazodone and trazodone to determine the risk during pregnancy. Animal studies have found some abnormalities in the fetus during maternal exposure to these agents. However, interpretation of the findings from animal studies in regard to human risk is unclear. The risk of nefazodone and trazodone to the fetus cannot be ruled out, and these agents should be prescribed during pregnancy only if the benefits outweigh the potential risk.

Trazodone has been found in breast milk, but it is not known whether nefazodone is excreted. It is recommended that women taking nefazodone or trazodone not breastfeed.

If you have any questions about this handout, please consult your physician.

INFORMATION ABOUT

SELECTIVE SEROTONIN REUPTAKE INHIBITORS (SSRIS)

FOR PATIENTS AND FAMILIES

- **Citalopram (Celexa)**
- **Escitalopram (Lexapro)**
- **Fluoxetine (Prozac)**
- **Fluvoxamine (Luvox)**
- **Paroxetine (Paxil, Paxil CR)**
- **Sertraline (Zoloft)**

The group of antidepressants known as **selective serotonin reuptake inhibitors** (SSRIs) includes the well-known drug **Prozac**. The term *SSRI* denotes the unique mechanism of action of these agents in the brain. It is hypothesized that diminished levels of neurotransmitters in the brain may cause depression and that depression may be the result of low levels of one or more neurotransmitters. One type of neurotransmitter in the brain is **serotonin.** If the depression is due to low levels of serotonin, enhancing the neurotransmission of serotonin may then treat the depression. SSRIs work by blocking the reuptake of serotonin back into brain cells (neurons) after it has been released, thereby preventing its breakdown. As more serotonin is made available, the brain undergoes changes that ultimately relieve depression. The lag time for the brain to normalize may explain why antidepressants may take weeks before their full effects are achieved.

The SSRI antidepressants are prescribed for depressive disorders, but they are also effective in treating a variety of other psychiatric disorders, including obsessive-compulsive disorder, anxiety disorders, eating disorders (bulimia nervosa and anorexia nervosa), premenstrual dysphoric disorder, panic disorder, and post-traumatic stress disorder.

The SSRIs are safer and easier to tolerate than the older antidepressants, such as the **monoamine oxidase inhibitors** (MAOIs) and **tricyclic antidepressants** (TCAs). The SSRIs have fewer side effects than the older antidepressants, and they are significantly safer in overdose. Fatal overdoses from SSRIs, although possible, are rare.

Currently, there are six SSRIs approved for use in the United States. Fluoxetine, fluvoxamine, and paroxetine (except Paxil CR) are available generically, whereas the others are marketed only under their brand. Citalopram, fluoxetine, paroxetine, and sertraline come in liquid dosage forms as well.

HOW SSRIs ARE PRESCRIBED

The dosage needed to treat acute depression is usually higher than the maintenance dose needed to prevent recurrence of depression. After acute depression has improved, it may be possible to reduce the dose of the antidepressant. The dosages of SSRIs for treatment of depression are generally lower than those for treatment of other psychiatric disorders. For example, the usual antidepressant dose for fluoxetine is 20 mg/day, whereas the recommended dose for treatment of bulimia nervosa is 60 mg/day. In Table 1, the usual dosage range and the maximum daily dose for SSRI antidepressants are listed.

Table 1. Selective Serotonin Reuptake Inhibitors: Usual Dosage Range and Maximum Daily Dose for Treatment of Depression

Generic name	Trade name	Usual dosage range, mg/day	Maximum total daily dose, mg
Citalopram	Celexa	20–40	40
Escitalopram	Lexapro	10–20	20
Fluoxetine	Prozac	20–40	80
Fluvoxamine	Luvox	100–200	300
Paroxetine	Paxil	20–50	50
Sertraline	Zoloft	50–100	200

PROPER USE OF YOUR MEDICATION

Storing Your Medication

- Keep your medication in a tamper-resistant vial and out of reach of children.
- Store your medication so as to keep it from excessive heat, moisture, and direct light.
- Keep your medication in its original prescription vial with the label intact to prevent others from inadvertently taking the medication.

Taking Your Medication

- Take your medication as instructed by your physician. Do not abruptly stop taking your antidepressant without consulting your physician. Discontinuation of your medication may result in relapse. SSRIs, like all antidepressants, may take up to 3 weeks to achieve full effect, and improvement may continue for 12 weeks
- If you miss a dose, take it as soon as possible. However, if it is near to the time of your next dose, skip the dose you missed and go back to your regular dosing schedule, but do not double-up the dose.
- These antidepressants may be taken with or without food. If an SSRI upsets your stomach, take it at mealtime.

Use of Alcohol and Other Medications

Individuals should refrain from using alcohol while taking antidepressants. Alcohol is a depressant and may exacerbate the depressive symptoms, and it may oppose the action of the antidepressant medication.

Certain medications, including over-the-counter medicines, may interact with the SSRI antidepressants. The drug interaction may *lower* the blood level of the affected drug and decrease its effectiveness; or, it may *elevate* the blood level of the affected drug and cause toxicity. There are some drugs when combined with the antidepressant may exacerbate some side effects. Inform your doctor of all the prescription and over-the-counter medications you are taking.

Patients taking SSRIs should not take an amino acid supplement called L-tryptophan, which is promoted for insomnia and depression. The combination may produce a central toxic reaction called **serotonin syndrome** (see "Possible Adverse Reactions"). Patients taking SSRIs should *never* take another type of antidepressant known as a **monoamine oxidase inhibitor**. The combination may produce severe elevation of blood pressure, fever, possible seizures, and even death. Furthermore, an SSRI should not be started within 2 weeks of discontinuing treatment with an MAOI; similarly, an MAOI should not be started within 2 weeks after stopping an SSRI, and longer for fluoxetine. If you have any questions or concerns with your medications, consult your physician or pharmacist.

POSSIBLE SIDE EFFECTS

- *Gastrointestinal side effects.* These side effects include nausea, diarrhea, cramping, dry mouth, heartburn, constipation, and gastrointestinal discomfort. Gastrointestinal side effects are more frequent at the higher dosages, but they will diminish after the first 2 weeks of therapy. If the dose is increased gradually, SSRI-induced gastrointestinal side effects may be minimized. Taking the antidepressant with meals may also reduce gastrointestinal distress. Patients taking paroxetine may benefit from the controlled-release tablets of paroxetine (**Paxil CR**), which may improve tolerability by reducing gastrointestinal side effects.
- *Anxiety, nervousness, and insomnia.* Patients taking SSRI antidepressants commonly complain of these arousing side effects. Patients may experience jitteriness, anxiety, restlessness, sleeplessness (insomnia), and irritability. Usually these side effects subside after 1–2 weeks. If insomnia is a problem, taking the antidepressant early in the day may offset this side effect. If this does not help, the physician may prescribe a hypnotic agent to help with sleep. **Trazodone**, a sedating antidepressant, is often prescribed briefly in low doses for insomnia. Also, trazodone may augment the response to SSRIs. The physician may prescribe other hypnotic agents as well, including diphenhydramine (Benadryl), a benzodiazepine such as **temazepam** (Restoril), **zolpidem** (Ambien), or **zaleplon** (Sonata).
- *Sedation and drowsiness.* For some patients, SSRIs may have the opposite effect and induce sedation, which is seen commonly with paroxetine. If daytime sedation is a problem, patients should take the antidepressant closer to bedtime.
- *Sexual dysfunction.* SSRIs may induce sexual dysfunction, including impotence, delayed ejaculation, diminished libido, and anorgasmia (inability to achieve orgasm). Although many patients may be hesitant to discuss their sexual problems, they are encouraged to do so with their doctor. The physician may suggest switching to another antidepressant with a lower incidence of inducing sexual dysfunction.
- *Weight changes and appetite.* Some patients may experience weight gain while taking SSRIs. However, in general, most of the SSRIs do not induce weight gain or induce only modest weight increases. Fluoxetine has been reported to suppress appetite, and some patients may lose weight. Generally, this side effect is brief, and fluoxetine is not a good appetite suppressant for patients on a diet.
- *Skin rash and sweating.* Up to 4% of the patients taking fluoxetine may develop a skin rash. Some rashes may have accompanied aches, joint pain, and elevated temperature. At the first sign of rash, the patient should discontinue the medication and contact his or her physician. Often, the patient's rash improves promptly when medication is discontinued, but the physician may prescribe an antihistamine such as **diphenhydramine** (Benadryl) to relieve the itch. Some patients taking fluoxetine may find that they perspire excessively. If excessive perspiration is problematic, an alternative is to switch to another antidepressant.

POSSIBLE ADVERSE REACTIONS

- *Suicide, violence, and fluoxetine.* When fluoxetine (Prozac) was first marketed in the United States, concerns were raised that depressed patients taking Prozac may have an increased risk of suicide. This association was made during early treatment with Prozac when it was reported that six patients had developed persistent and intense preoccupation with suicide. Other reports suggested that patients taking fluoxetine may injure themselves, as well as others. Since the original reports, several large studies failed to find any greater tendency for suicide or violence with fluoxetine than with other antidepressants. The studies indicated that suicidal behavior may be the result of the patient's underlying depression rather than from use of the antidepressant.

- *Seizures.* Rarely, seizures have occurred with the SSRIs at rates similar to those with other antidepressants but lower than those with tricyclic antidepressants. Caution must be exercised with use of antidepressants in patients with a history of seizure disorder.

- *Activation of mania or hypomania.* Use of SSRIs, as well as other antidepressants, may result in activation of a manic or hypomanic (less severe form of mania) episode for patients with bipolar disorder. Therefore, when these antidepressants are used in bipolar patient, the patient should be monitored closely for early signs of mania or hypomania.

- *Serotonin syndrome.* If SSRIs are combined with other medicines that increase serotonin, a reaction called **serotonin syndrome** may result. Medications that may potentiate SSRIs include MAOIs, L-tryptophan, psychostimulants such as amphetamines, and other antidepressants that enhance serotonin, including St. John's wort. Symptoms of serotonin syndrome include restlessness, confusion, tremors, twitching, loss of coordination, elevated body temperature, and loss of consciousness. When severe and untreated, serotonin syndrome may be fatal. Therefore, patients should check with their physician or pharmacist before self-medicating with any other medications, including nonprescription medicines.

- *Movement disorders.* Rarely, SSRI antidepressants cause movement disorders similar to those seen with antipsychotic medications. These movement disorders are known as **extrapyramidal symptoms** (EPS). One type of EPS is **akathisia**, which some patients may experience from SSRIs. Akathisia is described as an inner feeling of restlessness, expressed by constant pacing, inability to sit still, and nervousness. Usually, these reactions from SSRIs are mild and reversible when the dose is lowered.

PREGNANCY AND BREAST FEEDING

All the SSRIs are classified in **Category C** of the U.S. Food and Drug Administration (FDA) Pregnancy Risk Categories. They are given this classification because there are no clinical studies in women, nor is there adequate information, to determine the risk of these agents during pregnancy. Animal studies have found some abnormalities in the fetus during maternal exposure to these agents. However, interpretation of the findings from the animal studies in regard to human risk is unclear. The risk of SSRIs to the fetus cannot be ruled out, and these agents should be prescribed during pregnancy only if the benefits outweigh the potential risk.

Except for sertraline, SSRIs are excreted in human breast milk. It is not known whether, and if so in what amount, sertraline is excreted in breast milk. It is recommended that women taking SSRI antidepressants not breastfeed. The long-term effects from exposure of SSRI antidepressants to the developing infant are unknown.

If you have any questions about this handout, please consult your physician.

INFORMATION ABOUT

TRICYCLIC AND TETRACYCLIC ANTIDEPRESSANTS (TCAs)

FOR PATIENTS AND FAMILIES

○ **Amitriptyline (Elavil)**

○ **Amoxapine (Asendin)**

○ **Clomipramine (Anafranil)**

○ **Desipramine (Norpramin)**

○ **Doxepin (Sinequan)**

○ **Imipramine (Tofranil)**

○ **Maprotiline (Ludiomil)**

○ **Nortriptyline (Pamelor)**

○ **Protriptyline (Vivactil)**

○ **Trimipramine (Surmontil)**

The **tricyclic and tetracyclic antidepressants** are so-called because they have three-ring and four-ring chemical structures, respectively. These antidepressants are remarkably similar and are commonly lumped together and referred to simply as *tricyclic antidepressants,* or **TCAs**, of which **Elavil** (amitriptyline) is the best known. For convenience, this handout shall refer to the tricyclic and tetracyclic antidepressants as TCAs.

The TCAs are not as widely prescribed for treatment of depression as they once were. Physicians are more likely to select antidepressants with fewer side effects than the TCAs—for example, a selective serotonin reuptake inhibitor (SSRI) such as fluoxetine (Prozac). TCAs are, however, effective antidepressants and have been the standard for treatment of major depression against which other antidepressants are measured.

The primary indication for TCAs is for treatment of major depression. Other U.S. Food and Drug Administration (FDA)–approved uses include treatment of anxiety (doxepin), childhood enuresis (imipramine), and obsessive-compulsive disorder (clomipramine). Because TCAs have a broad range of action, these compounds are prescribed for non-FDA-approved, but common, uses in other areas of medicine. (The FDA's approved indications only limit how manufacturers may market their products but do not restrict how physicians may prescribe them.) TCAs are commonly used in treatment of migraine headaches, with other analgesics for pain management, sleep disorder, panic disorder, eating disorder (bulimia), and peptic ulcer disease.

It is hypothesized that diminished levels of neurotransmitters in the brain may cause depression and that depression may be the result of low levels of one or more of neurotransmitters. TCAs work by increasing the level of neurotransmitters—principally **norepinephrine** and **serotonin**. Increasing the level of these neurotransmitters perhaps facilitates the brain in undergoing changes that ultimately relieve the depression. The lag time for the brain to normalize may explain why antidepressants may take weeks before their full effects are achieved.

The 10 TCAs marketed in the United States are listed at the beginning of this handout under their generic and common brand names.

HOW THESE ANTIDEPRESSANTS ARE PRESCRIBED

The dosages for TCAs used for treating depression vary with each antidepressant. Starting with a low dose and then increasing the dose gradually may reduce the side effects of the TCAs and make them more tolerable. The antidepressant effect usually occurs when the dose is within the *therapeutic range*. Physicians may order blood levels to help gauge when the dose is within the therapeutic range.

When possible, a single, convenient bedtime dose is administered to minimize daytime sedation and other bothersome side effects. If the patient cannot tolerate a single dose, the antidepressant may be taken in divided doses. Generally, lower dosages are needed for adolescent and elderly patients. It may take several weeks before the patient feels any significant response.

PROPER USE OF YOUR MEDICATION

Storing Your Medication

- Keep your medication in a tamper-resistant vial and out of reach of children. Acute overdosage with TCAs is extremely dangerous for infants and children.
- Store your medication so as to keep it from excessive heat, moisture, and direct light.
- Keep your medication in its original prescription vial with the label intact to prevent others from taking the medication inadvertently.

Taking Your Medication

- Take your medication exactly as instructed by your physician. Do not abruptly stop taking your medication without telling your physician. Abrupt discontinuation of your medication may result in unpleasant withdrawal symptoms and relapse of symptoms. TCAs should be decreased gradually before discontinuation.
- TCAs, like all antidepressants, may take several weeks to achieve their full effect.
- If you miss a dose, take it as soon as possible. However, if it is near the time of your next dose, skip the dose you missed and go back to your regular dosing schedule, but do not double-up the dose.
- Your antidepressant may be taken with or without food. If it upsets your stomach, take it at mealtime.

Use of Alcohol and Other Medications

Individuals should refrain from consuming alcohol while taking antidepressants. Alcohol is a depressant and may oppose the action of the antidepressant.

Certain medications, including over-the-counter medicines, may interact with TCAs and should not be taken concomitantly. The drug interaction may *lower* the blood level of the affected drug and decrease the drug's effectiveness; or, it may *elevate* the blood level of the affected drug and cause toxicity. When certain drugs are combined with TCAs, they may exacerbate some side effects. Inform your physician of all prescription and over-the-counter medications you are taking. If you have questions about your medications, consult your physician or pharmacist.

TCAs should *never* be used in combination with **monoamine oxidase inhibitor** (MAOI) antidepressants. This combination can precipitate a dangerous reaction (see "Possible Adverse Reactions").

POSSIBLE SIDE EFFECTS

Patients should not become unduly alarmed if they experience some bothersome side effects from these antidepressants, especially shortly after beginning therapy. These side effects usually subside as the individual becomes better adjusted to the medication. If the side effects become intolerable or persist, a reduction in the dosage may be necessary.

- *Sedation.* This is the most frequent complaint from patients taking TCAs. Taking the TCA antidepressant in a single bedtime dose, if possible, may minimize daytime sedation. Usually, patients develop tolerance to the sedative effects of TCAs.
- *Anticholinergic side effects.* When TCAs interfere with the part of the nervous system that regulates those body functions—the cholinergic system—it produces unwanted side effects. Hence, drugs that inhibit the function of the cholinergic nervous system produce **anticholinergic side effects.** These side effects include dry mouth, blurred vision, impaired accommodation (disturbance of the eye muscles so that it becomes difficult to adjust to nearby objects), constipation, urinary retention, and hesitancy, dizziness, and palpitations. Furthermore, excessive anticholinergic action can produce confusion and memory impairment, especially in elderly patients.

  Physicians may prescribe **bethanechol** (25–50 mg/day) to combat the anticholinergic side effects of urinary retention and hesitancy. Eating a high-fiber diet, increasing fluid intake, and using a bulk laxative, such as Metamucil, or a stool softener may prevent constipation.

  In patients with a history of narrow-angle glaucoma or increased intraocular pressure, TCAs must be used with caution. In patients with urinary hesitancy, especially men with enlarged prostates, anticholinergic effects of TCAs may exacerbate the problem.
- *Sexual dysfunction.* TCAs may induce sexual dysfunction, including impotence, delayed ejaculation, diminished libido, and anorgasmia (inability to achieve orgasm). Although many patients may be hesitant to discuss their sexual problems, they are encouraged to do so with their doctor. The physician may suggest switching to another antidepressant with a lower incidence of inducing sexual dysfunction.
- *Weight gain.* Patients taking TCAs may experience weight gain, which is especially common with clomipramine treatment.
- *Orthostatic hypotension.* Low blood pressure due to a postural change is known as **orthostatic hypotension**. TCAs may oppose the body's ability to elevate blood pressure when there is a change in position. If the blood pressure cannot elevate in time to compensate for the change in position as the individual rises from a lying or sitting position, orthostatic hypotension ensues. As a result, the individual feels light-headed and dizzy, has a rapid heart rate, and may faint and fall. The patient can avoid or minimize orthostatic hypotension by rising slowly to allow the blood pressure to adjust. Elderly patients and patients taking larger doses may be more susceptible to orthostatic hypotension and should be cautious of this side effect.
- *Other possible side effects.* Dizziness, nasal congestion, muscle twitching, tremors, confusion, nervousness, palpitations, excessive perspiration, fatigue, and headache are also possible. If any of these side effects persist or are intolerable, discuss the problem with your physician.

> **Warning**:   TCAs may cause drowsiness and dizziness. Patients must exercise caution when engaging in daily activities that require mental alertness, such as operating a motor vehicle. It is recommended that patients do not engage in hazardous tasks until they are reasonably certain that their medication does not adversely affect their performance or impair their judgment.

POSSIBLE ADVERSE REACTIONS

- *Seizures.* TCAs can lower seizure threshold and potentially precipitate seizures in susceptible individuals, especially those with a history of seizure disorder. Clomipramine and maprotiline are associated with a higher risk of seizures, especially with overdose.
- *Adverse drug reaction.* The MAOI antidepressants, such as **phenelzine** (Nardil), **tranylcypromine** (Parnate), **isocarboxazid** (Marplan), and **selegiline** (Eldepryl), should *never* be taken with TCAs. Moreover, they should not be used within 14 days before or after treatment with a TCA. This combination may produce a severe reaction that results in sweating, flushing, confusion, restlessness, elevated temperature, and possibly seizures. Complications from severely elevated blood pressure (**hypertensive crisis)** may be fatal.

- *Caution in patients with cardiovascular disease.* In patients with cardiovascular disease, and especially those with a history of arrhythmias, coronary artery disease, congestive heart failure, or a recent heart attack, TCAs must be prescribed with caution, if at all. TCAs may alter the electrical conduction of the heart and prolong conduction time. These effects may produce arrhythmias and rapid heart rate. A rapid heart rate may cause chest pains or precipitate a heart attack in patients with coronary heart disease.
- *Overdose.* Overdosage with TCAs is extremely dangerous, and these antidepressants have been the leading cause of death from intentional overdoses. Cardiac arrhythmias from disturbances of heart rhythm are the most frequent cause of death. TCA overdose is a medical emergency that requires immediate, aggressive intervention and removal of the antidepressant from the patient's stomach before significant amounts are absorbed.

PREGNANCY AND BREAST FEEDING

Amitriptyline, imipramine, and nortriptyline are associated with congenital malformations, and they are classified in **Category D** of the FDA Pregnancy Risk Categories. In this category, there is evidence that these antidepressants are associated with human fetal risk, and they should be avoided during pregnancy.

Amoxapine, clomipramine, desipramine, doxepin, protriptyline, and trimipramine are classified in **Category C** of the FDA Pregnancy Risk Categories. There are no controlled studies with these antidepressants during pregnancy from which to determine the extent of human fetal risk. However, in animal studies, at very high doses, these antidepressants produced harmful effects on the fetus. The interpretation of findings from animal studies in regard to human risk is unclear. Only when the benefits absolutely outweigh the risks should these TCAs be prescribed during pregnancy.

Small amounts of TCAs are excreted into breast milk. Women who are taking TCAs should not breastfeed. There may be harmful effects if infant absorbs the antidepressant.

If you have any questions about this handout, please consult your physician.

INFORMATION ABOUT

VENLAFAXINE (EFFEXOR AND EFFEXOR XR)

FOR PATIENTS AND FAMILIES

Venlafaxine (Effexor and Effexor XR) is an effective antidepressant for treatment of different types of depressive disorders, especially refractory and melancholia depression. Another important use of venlafaxine is in the treatment of anxiety disorders. The U.S. Food and Drug Administration (FDA) approved venlafaxine for the treatment of depression and generalized anxiety disorder. For patients diagnosed with both depression and anxiety, venlafaxine may be effective in treating mixed symptoms. Venlafaxine is also prescribed for obsessive-compulsive disorder, attention-deficit/hyperactivity disorder in children and adults, and posttraumatic stress disorder.

It is hypothesized that diminished levels of neurotransmitters in the brain may cause depression, and depression may be the result of low levels of one or more neurotransmitters. Venlafaxine's antidepressant effect may be related to its action in increasing the levels of neurotransmitters. As more neurotransmitters are made available, the brain undergoes changes that ultimately relieve depression. The lag time for the brain to normalize explains why antidepressants, including venlafaxine, may take weeks before their full effects are achieved.

Venlafaxine is marketed under its trade names **Effexor** and **Effexor XR;** there is no generic substitution for this antidepressant. Effexor XR, the extended-release formulation of venlafaxine, may be taken once a day. With the convenience of once-a-day dosing and an improved side-effect profile, physicians prefer prescribing Effexor XR over Effexor for their patients.

Effexor is available in 25-, 37.5-, 50-, 75-, and 100-mg tablets. Effexor XR is available in 37.5-, 75-, and 150-mg capsules.

HOW VENLAFAXINE IS PRESCRIBED

The recommended starting dosage for immediate-release venlafaxine (Effexor) is 75 mg/day, taken in two or three divided doses (e.g., 25 mg three times a day, or 37.5 mg twice a day). The dosage may be increased, depending on tolerability and clinical response, by 75 mg/day at 4-day intervals, to a maximum total daily dose of 225 mg.

Extended-release venlafaxine (Effexor XR) may be taken in a single dose. Patients treated at a therapeutic dose with immediate-release venlafaxine may be switched to the extended-release form (e.g., 37.5 mg Effexor two times a day to 75 mg Effexor XR once a day). However, today physicians usually prescribe Effexor XR rather than Effexor. Effexor XR is started at 37.5 mg once a day, and the dosage is increased in increments of 75 mg/day at 4-day intervals. For treatment of depression, most patients respond to dosages in the range of 75 to 225 mg/day.

PROPER USE OF YOUR MEDICATION

Storing Your Medication

- Keep your medication in a tamper-resistant vial and out of reach of children.
- Store your medication so as to keep it from excessive heat, moisture, and direct light.

- Keep your medication in its original prescription vial with the label intact to prevent others from taking the medication inadvertently.

Taking Your Medication

- Take your medication as instructed by your physician. Do not abruptly stop taking your medication without consulting your physician. Discontinuation of your medication may result in relapse. When venlafaxine is being discontinued, your physician may need to decrease the dose gradually to prevent withdrawal symptoms. Venlafaxine, like all antidepressants, may take several weeks to achieve its full effect.
- If you miss a dose, take it as soon as possible. However, if it is near the time of your next dose, skip the dose you missed and go back to your regular dosing schedule, but do not double-up the dose.
- It is best to take venlafaxine with food.
- Effexor XR should be swallowed whole and not crushed or chewed.

Use of Alcohol and Other Medications

Individuals should refrain from alcohol consumption while taking antidepressants. Alcohol is a depressant and may oppose the action of the antidepressant medication.

Certain medications, including over-the-counter medicines, may interact with venlafaxine. The drug interaction may *lower* the blood level of the affected drug and decrease the drug's effectiveness; or, it may *elevate* the blood level of the affected drug and cause toxicity. When certain drugs are combined with venlafaxine, they may exacerbate some side effects. Inform your physician of all prescription and over-the-counter medications you are taking.

Patients taking venlafaxine should *never* take a **monoamine oxidase inhibitor** (MAOI) antidepressant concomitantly. MAOI antidepressants include **phenelzine** (Nardil), **tranylcypromine** (Parnate), and **isocarboxazid** (Marplan). The combination may precipitate severe elevation of blood pressure, fever, and possible seizures. The reaction may be fatal if medical treatment is not provided to the patient immediately.

POSSIBLE SIDE EFFECTS

- *Insomnia and nervousness.* These side effects are the most frequent complaints from patients after starting treatment with venlafaxine. Patients with insomnia may benefit from taking Effexor XR in a single dose in the morning. If this does not alleviate the problem, the physician may prescribe a hypnotic agent to help with sleep. **Trazodone**, a sedating antidepressant, is often prescribed briefly in low doses for sleep. Also, trazodone may augment the response to venlafaxine. Other hypnotic agents that may prove useful include **diphenhydramine** (Benadryl), a benzodiazepine such as **temazepam** (Restoril), **zolpidem** (Ambien), or **zaleplon** (Sonata). If the patient feels nervous and jittery from venlafaxine, the physician may start with a lower dose and then increase the dose slowly.
- *Drowsiness, tiredness, and dizziness.* These side effects are usually self-limiting as the patient becomes adjusted to the medication. If they persist, it may indicate the need for a lower dose. Patients must exercise caution and refrain from performing hazardous tasks, including driving an automobile, until they are certain that venlafaxine does not adversely affect their ability to engage in those activities.
- *Gastrointestinal (GI) side effects.* Dry mouth, nausea, and constipation are common GI complaints. Take venlafaxine at mealtime to reduce nausea. These side effects usually subside over time.
- *Change in appetite and weight loss.* Some patients taking venlafaxine may experience decreased appetite and weight loss. In an underweight, depressed patient, this may be an undesirable result. If appetite change and weight loss are problematic, the patient should consult with the physician.
- *Sexual dysfunction.* Venlafaxine may induce sexual dysfunction, including impotence, delayed ejaculation, diminished libido, and anorgasmia (inability to achieve orgasm). Although some patients may be hesitant to talk about their sexual problems, they are encouraged to discuss their concerns with their doctor. The physician may suggest switching to another antidepressant with a lower incidence of sexual dysfunction.

- *Withdrawal symptoms.* Patients who have been taking venlafaxine for any extended period should not abruptly discontinue their medication. They may experience withdrawal symptoms such as nervousness, dizziness, flulike symptoms, and depression. Discontinuation of venlafaxine should be done gradually, decreasing the dose slowly before stopping.

> **Warning**: Venlafaxine may cause drowsiness and dizziness. Patients must exercise caution when engaging in daily activities that require mental alertness, such as operating a motor vehicle. It is recommended that patients do not engage in hazardous tasks until they are reasonably certain that their medication does not adversely affect their performance or impair their judgment.

POSSIBLE ADVERSE REACTIONS

- *Elevated blood pressure.* Venlafaxine may elevate blood pressure, even in patients without preexisting high blood pressure. The incidence of elevated blood pressure induced by venlafaxine may be as high as 5%, but this rate may be lower with the extended-release form. Usually, blood pressure is slightly elevated without the need to discontinue medication. Occasionally, however, blood pressure may be moderately elevated, and the venlafaxine will have to be discontinued. The elevated blood pressure did not result in a life-threatening sequela once the antidepressant was discontinued. Apparently, patients with hypertension are not necessarily more prone to greater increases in blood pressure from venlafaxine as compared with patients without preexisting hypertension. Pretreatment blood pressure should be established before starting venlafaxine and monitored routinely while taking venlafaxine, especially when the dosage is greater than 225 mg/day. Venlafaxine should be used cautiously in patients with hypertension, and blood pressure should be monitored more frequently.
- *Serotonin syndrome.* When venlafaxine is taken with other medications that boost **serotonin**, the combination may potentially produce excessive serotonin and overstimulation of the central nervous system. This condition is known as **serotonin syndrome,** which consists of restlessness, confusion, flushing, sweating, shaking of the hands, and involuntary jerking of the body. If the medications causing the problem are not discontinued immediately, it may lead to further complications. Patients should be aware of the medications that may put them at risk for serotonin syndrome. MAOIs should *never* be combined with venlafaxine. Selective serotonin reuptake inhibitor (SSRI) antidepressants, such as fluoxetine (Prozac), should be prescribed cautiously and at lower doses when combined with venlafaxine. Patients should not self-medicate with St. John's wort, an over-the-counter medicine promoted to help depression. Patients should consult their physician or pharmacist if they have questions about their medications.
- *Mania and hypomania.* In patients with bipolar disorder, when the depressive phase of the illness is being treated with antidepressants, there is a risk that the medication will precipitate mania or hypomania (a less severe form of mania). Although the incidence of mania-hypomania switching is very low during treatment with venlafaxine, individuals with a history of bipolar illness should be aware of this reaction.

PREGNANCY AND BREAST FEEDING

Venlafaxine is classified in **Category C** of the FDA Pregnancy Risk Categories. It is given this classification because there are no clinical studies, or there is inadequate information, on the use of venlafaxine in women to determine the risk during pregnancy. Animal studies have found some abnormalities in the fetus during maternal exposure to venlafaxine. However, interpretation of the findings from animal studies in regard to human risks is unclear. The risk of venlafaxine cannot be ruled out, and it should be prescribed during pregnancy only if the benefits outweigh the potential risk.

Venlafaxine is excreted in human breastmilk. Women taking venlafaxine should not breastfeed.

If you have any questions about this handout, please consult your physician.

INFORMATION ABOUT

CARBAMAZEPINE (TEGRETOL AND TEGRETOL-XR) AND OXCARBAZEPINE (TRILEPTAL)

FOR PATIENTS AND FAMILIES

Carbamazepine (Tegretol, Tegretol-XR) and **oxcarbazepine** (Trileptal) are anticonvulsants used to treat and prevent seizures. However, in psychiatry, these agents are used to treat and prevent mania and depression in bipolar disorder. When anticonvulsants such as carbamazepine and oxcarbazepine are prescribed for treatment of mood disorders, they are referred to as *mood stabilizers*.

It is thought that anticonvulsants work for both seizures and mania because they control and stabilize *"kindling,"* which consists of unstable, repetitive electrical stimulations of the brain. Once triggered, either by psychological stress or by injury to the susceptible area of the brain, kindling can set off the nervous system, which may result in seizures or manic behavior, depending on the individual's susceptibility. Perhaps this mechanism of action, albeit oversimplified, can help explain why some anticonvulsants are effective for treating seizures and mood disorders.

Carbamazepine is available in 100-mg chewable tablets and 200-mg tablets. Commonly known by the brand **Tegretol**, it is available and dispensed mostly in generic tablets. It is available in oral suspension in a concentration of 100 mg/5 mL (teaspoonful). Tegretol also comes in an extended-release tablet, called **Tegretol-XR**, which is available in 100-, 200-, and 400-mg strengths.

The chemical structure of oxcarbazepine (**Trileptal**) is very similar to that of carbamazepine, and the two agents share similar pharmacologic actions. Oxcarbazepine comes in 100-, 300-, and 600-mg tablets, but it is not available in a generic equivalent. Oxcarbazepine is also available in an oral suspension in a concentration of 300 mg/5 mL.

HOW THESE MEDICATIONS ARE PRESCRIBED

The starting dose for carbamazepine is usually 200 mg two or three times a day (400–600 mg/day), and the dosage is increased in increments of 200 mg/day every 3–5 days until clinical response is achieved or until adverse effects preclude higher dosing. Regular carbamazepine can be switched to the extended-release preparation by administering the total daily dose in two divided doses with the extended-release tablets. For most people, the maintenance dosage of carbamazepine for mood stabilization is between 600 and 1,600 mg/day.

The usual starting dose for oxcarbazepine is 300 mg two times a day (600 mg/day), and the maintenance dosage is between 600 and 2,400 mg/day.

Blood Tests Are Necessary

To determine that the dose of carbamazepine or oxcarbazepine is adequate, your doctor may order blood levels for the drug. Levels are repeated more frequently when the medication is being started, and periodically thereafter when the dose is stabilized. In addition, because carbamazepine is associated with a serious, but rare, adverse reaction (**aplastic anemia**; see "Possible Adverse Reactions"), your doctor may order a complete blood cell count (CBC) that may be repeated periodically during treatment to monitor for this potentially hazardous reaction.

PROPER USE OF YOUR MEDICATION

Storing Your Medication

- Keep your medication in a tamper-resistant vial or bottle and out of reach of children. Overdosage of carbamazepine or oxcarbazepine is very dangerous, particularly for young children.
- Store your medication so as to keep it from excessive heat, moisture, and direct light.
- Keep the medication in its original prescription vial with the prescription label intact to prevent others from taking the medication inadvertently.
- Do not use the medication past the expiration date on the prescription label.

Taking Your Medication

- If you miss a dose, take it as soon as possible. However, if it is 1–2 hours before your next dose, skip the dose you missed and go back to your regular dosing schedule, but do not double-up on the dose.
- Carbamazepine and oxcarbazepine may be taken with food without affecting their absorption. If the medication upsets your stomach, take it with food.
- If you are taking an extended-release tablet of carbamazepine, take the tablet whole; do not cut or crush the tablet.
- If you are taking carbamazepine or oxcarbazepine in the suspension form, shake the bottle thoroughly. Measure the quantity as specified on your prescription label. The concentration of carbamazepine suspension comes in 100 mg/5 mL (1 teaspoonful). For example, a 300-mg dose requires 15 mL (3 teaspoonfuls). Oxcarbazepine in the oral suspension is 300 mg/5 mL. A 600-mg dose, for example, requires 10 mL (2 teaspoonfuls).

Use of Alcohol and Other Medications

It is recommended that patients not consume alcohol when taking carbamazepine or oxcarbazepine. Alcohol may significantly increase the sedative effects of these medications, so that they may experience greater drowsiness and loss of coordination. In addition, alcohol may affect the metabolism of these drugs, and this may alter their blood levels and effectiveness. Before consuming alcohol, consult with your physician.

A number of drugs can affect the metabolism of carbamazepine or oxcarbazepine and, ultimately, their blood levels. As a result, the metabolism of some drugs can be affected by carbamazepine or oxcarbazepine and increase or decrease the blood levels of the drugs. When the drug level is *elevated*, toxicity may result, and when the drug level is *lowered*, the effectiveness may be decreased. You should inform your physician of all the prescription and over-the-counter medications you are taking. If you have questions or concerns, consult your physician or pharmacist.

There are several significant drug interactions with carbamazepine or oxcarbazepine the patient should be aware of. Carbamazepine and oxcarbazepine may result in lowering the level of **oral contraceptives** (birth-control pills), decreasing their effectiveness in preventing contraception. Carbamazepine may lower blood levels of **warfarin** (Coumadin), an oral anticoagulant, the anticonvulsants **phenytoin** (Dilantin) and **lamotrigine** (Lamictal), **tricyclic antidepressants**, and the antibiotic **doxycycline,** *decreasing* their effectiveness. Drugs that *increase* levels of carbamazepine include the anti-ulcer drug **cimetidine** (Tagamet); **phenobarbital;** some antidepressants, including **fluoxetine** (Prozac) and **fluvoxamine** (Luvox); and the antibiotics **erythromycin** and **clarithromycin** (Biaxin). Increased levels of carbamazepine may result in toxicity.

POSSIBLE SIDE EFFECTS

Most side effects from carbamazepine or oxcarbazepine are usually temporary and are generally easy to reverse when the dose is decreased or when the individual becomes adjusted to the medication.

- *Dizziness.* Usually, the patient adjusts to this side effect from carbamazepine or oxcarbazepine, but if it persists the dose may need to be lowered.
- *Drowsiness.* As the patient adjusts to the medication after the first week, drowsiness usually will not be bothersome, but the dose may need to be reduced if the drowsiness persists.
- *Loss of coordination, clumsiness, and confusion.* At higher doses, carbamazepine and oxcarbazepine may cause some of these side effects, which usually subside when the dose is reduced.
- *Nausea and vomiting.* Nausea, sometimes accompanied by vomiting, is a common complaint and generally occurs more often with carbamazepine than with oxcarbazepine. These side effects may be minimized by increasing the dose gradually or by decreasing the dose when they occur. Carbamazepine and oxcarbazepine should be taken with food.
- *Visual disturbance.* At high doses of carbamazepine and oxcarbazepine, the patient may complain of visual disturbance, such as blurred vision or jerky eye movements (nystagmus). Notify your physician when your experience visual disturbance, and do not operate a motor vehicle under these conditions.
- *Decreased sodium levels.* Oxcarbazepine, and carbamazepine to a lesser extent, may lower sodium blood levels (**hyponatremia**). This effect generally occurs during the first 3 months of treatment. In the cases reported, there were no severe results. However, if the patient is also taking a diuretic that lowers sodium, the physician should check sodium levels more frequently during the first 3 months of treatment.

> **Warning.** Carbamazepine and oxcarbazepine may cause drowsiness and sedation and impair physical coordination and mental alertness. Until you are sure that these side effects will not impair your ability to perform daily tasks, it important to avoid potentially dangerous activities, such as driving a car or operating machinery.

POSSIBLE ADVERSE REACTIONS

An adverse reaction to carbamazepine or oxcarbazepine is very rare, but when it occurs it may be serious and sometimes fatal. Patients should be aware of these potential risks and report any signs of abnormality to their physician.

- *Agranulocytosis.* This rare reaction reported with carbamazepine, but not with oxcarbazepine, results in a sudden drop in white blood cell (WBC) count. Levels of a particular type of WBCs, called **granulocytes**, which are important in fighting infections, are decreased; the medical term for this condition is **agranulocytosis**, or "without granulocytes." The risk of developing agranulocytosis is very low. Early detection and discontinuation of carbamazepine will result in complete recovery. Early warning signs of infection, including sore throat, malaise, and fever, should be reported to the physician if these symptoms persist.
- *Aplastic anemia.* A rare and potentially fatal adverse reaction is **aplastic anemia**, a condition in which the bone marrow stops producing white and red blood cells, including platelets (important for clotting). The risk of aplastic anemia from carbamazepine is extremely rare. If it occurs, the individual may develop infections from a low number of WBCs, anemia from a low number of red blood cells, and bleeding abnormalities from a low number of platelets. Usually physicians order pretreatment tests to evaluate blood cell count before starting carbamazepine treatment. Some physicians repeat blood count tests annually, whereas others may not because carbamazepine-induced aplastic anemia is so rare. More importantly, physicians instruct their patients to report any abnormal signs, including early signs of infection, such as fever and sore throat, bruising, weakness, and fatigue. The physician may then order blood tests to rule out aplastic anemia.

- *Abnormal liver function.* Occasionally, carbamazepine and oxcarbazepine cause elevation of liver enzymes. When enzymes are mildly elevated, this generally does not present any serious consequence, but liver function should be monitored more closely, because the enzyme levels usually return to normal. However, if levels of liver enzyme are persistently elevated or reach three times the normal level, drug treatment must be terminated. On rare occasions, carbamazepine has been reported to cause jaundice, in which yellowing occurs in the skin and may be noticeable in the whites of the eyes. This condition is caused by excessive bilirubin, a bile pigment, in the blood that cannot be removed properly from circulation because of diminished liver function. These reactions are usually reversed when carbamazepine or oxcarbazepine treatment is terminated.

PREGNANCY AND BREAST FEEDING

Carbamazepine is in **Category D** of the FDA Pregnancy Risk Categories. Carbamazepine may cause birth defects when it is administered during pregnancy, especially in the first trimester. Carbamazepine should not be taken during pregnancy. Carbamazepine-associated birth defects include head and facial abnormalities, developmental delays, and spinal cord and neural tube defects (**spina bifida**).

Oxcarbazepine is in **Category C.** It has not been sufficiently studied to conclude the safety of its use during pregnancy. Currently, there are insufficient data available to know the exact risks of oxcarbazepine to the woman and fetus. It has been shown that oxcarbazapine may induce fetal abnormalities in animal reproduction studies. Because oxcarbazepine is closely related in structure to carbamazepine, there is concern that oxcarbazepine may present some risks to the fetus. The need for the medication during pregnancy must be carefully weighed against the potential risks of the drug.

Carbamazepine and oxcarbazepine, and their metabolites, are excreted in breast milk. Women should not breastfeed when taking these medications because of the potential for harm to the infant when the drug is ingested.

If you have questions about this handout, please consult your physician.

INFORMATION ABOUT

DIVALPROEX (DEPAKOTE AND DEPAKOTE ER) AND VALPROIC ACID (DEPAKENE)

FOR PATIENTS AND FAMILIES

Divalproex (Depakote, Depakote ER) and **valproic acid** (Depakene) are anticonvulsants used for the treatment and prevention of seizure disorders. In psychiatry, divalproex and valproic acid are used in treating mania and depression of bipolar disorder. The U.S. Food and Drug Administration (FDA) approved divalproex, but not valproic acid, for treating acute mania in bipolar disorder. When anticonvulsants such as divalproex and valproic acid are used to stabilize moods in individuals diagnosed with bipolar disorder or manic-depressive illness, they are referred to as *mood stabilizers*.

It is thought that anticonvulsants control seizures and mania because they stabilize "kindling," which consists of unstable, repetitive electrical stimulations of the brain. Once triggered, either by psychological stress or by injury to the susceptible area of the brain, kindling can set off the nervous system, and this may result in seizures or manic behavior, depending on how susceptible the individual is. Perhaps this mechanism of action, albeit oversimplified, may explain why some anticonvulsants are effective for treating seizures and mood disorders.

Divalproex is a delayed-release formulation of valproic acid. Both medications have the same active ingredient; the difference is in the formulation of divalproex. Once ingested, divalproex is converted to valproic acid. For the sake of simplicity, and where applicable, we shall refer to divalproex and valproic acid as **valproate** in this handout.

Divalproex comes in tablets of 125-, 250-, and 500-mg strengths, and in a capsule form (**Depakote Sprinkle**) that can be pulled apart and mixed with food. Divalproex is also available in extended-release tablets (**Depakote ER**) that may be taken once a day. It is available in 250- and 500-mg tablets. Divalproex is marketed in the United States under the trade names Depakote and Depakote ER. Currently, generic equivalents are not available for divalproex.

Valproic acid comes in a gel capsule, only in 250-mg strength, and in a syrup form. The syrup contains 250 mg of valproic acid per 5 mL (1 teaspoonful). Valproic acid is marketed under the brand name **Depakene** but is available generically from various manufacturers.

HOW DIVALPROEX AND VALPROIC ACID ARE PRESCRIBED

Divalproex is prescribed more frequently than valproic acid because it does not irritate the stomach as much as valproic acid and may be dosed less frequently. The recommended starting dose of divalproex for treatment of acute mania is 250 mg three times a day, and the dosage is increased rapidly over the course of 3–7 days to achieve the desired clinical response or until the drug reaches therapeutic blood levels (see "Blood Tests Are Necessary"). Most patients achieve therapeutic levels at a dosage of 1,200–1,500 mg/day administered in two divided doses. Taking a larger dose at bedtime rather than in the morning may minimize daytime sedation. The dosage for valproic acid is the same as for divalproex. However, valproic acid must be taken more frequently—three or four times daily. Patients who are stabilized on valproic acid may be switched to divalproex by administering the same total daily dose but converting the dosing to a twice-daily schedule.

In the hospital, physicians may prescribe a divalproex "loading dose" to treat acute mania. With this strategy, the physician uses a large dose of divalproex immediately and then slowly tapers the dose. A loading-dose strategy has been shown to be effective in producing a rapid response in some patients, but the patient must be carefully monitored.

The dose for Depakote ER is the same as for Depakote, but the ER tablets can be taken in a single daily dose, preferably close to bedtime. The recommended starting dose for Depakote ER is 500 mg once a day for 1 week, and then the dose is increased to 1,000 mg taken once a day. Further increases may be made in 250- or 500-mg increments as needed.

Blood Tests Are Necessary

Valproate blood levels help the physician gauge the patient's dosing. A plasma valproate level from 50 to 125 µg/mL is usually considered an effective level; higher levels may be associated with side effects and toxicity. However, it is the patient's clinical response that ultimately determines the dose. Valproate levels are usually obtained weekly for the first 3 weeks until a stable dose is achieved, and then monthly for the next 3 months; thereafter, most physicians order a level every 3–6 months.

Because valproate is metabolized in the liver, blood tests to evaluate the patient's liver function are routinely done before valproate is started. Additionally, the physician may obtain a complete blood count (CBC), including a platelet count, before starting the medication. While you are taking valproate, your physician may repeat these tests periodically to monitor progress.

PROPER USE OF YOUR MEDICATION

Storing Your Medication

- Keep your medication in a tamper-resistant vial and away from children. Overdosage of valproate is very dangerous, particularly for young children.
- Store your medication so as to keep it from excessive heat, moisture, and direct light. Valproic acid capsules are susceptible to breakdown when exposed to heat and moisture.
- Keep the medication in its original prescription vial with the prescription label intact to prevent others from taking the medication inadvertently.
- Do not use the medication past the expiration date on the prescription label.

Taking Your Medication

- If you miss a dose of divalproex or valproic acid, take it as soon as possible. However, if it is 1–2 hours before your next dose, skip the dose you missed and go back to your regular dosing schedule, but do not double the dose. If you miss your daily dose of Depakote ER, take it as soon as possible, but if it is 2–3 hours before your next dose, skip the missed dose and go back to your regular dosing schedule.
- Swallow the tablets or capsules whole; do not chew, cut, or crush them.
- You may take valproate with food if the medicine upsets your stomach.
- If you are taking valproic acid syrup, measure the quantity as specified on your prescription label. It comes in a concentration of 250 mg/5 mL (1 teaspoonful). For example, a dose of 1,000 mg requires 20 mL (4 teaspoonfuls).
- If you have diabetes and must check your urine ketones, it is important that you know that valproate may interfere with urine tests for ketones and produce false positive results. It is suggested that you consult your pharmacist.

Use of Alcohol and Other Medications

No medication, including alcohol and over-the-counter medications, should be taken with valproate without your physician's approval. Alcohol may alter the metabolism of valproate and reduce its effectiveness. Moreover, the sedative effects of alcohol and valproate are greater when the two are taken together. Operating a motor vehicle under these conditions is extremely dangerous.

You should be aware that certain drugs alter the metabolism of valproate, which may decrease or increase the blood levels of valproate. When valproate blood levels are lowered, it may reduce its effectiveness, and when levels are increased, toxicity may result. For example, the antibiotic erythromycin may increase valproate blood levels and result in valproate toxicity. If you have questions or concerns about possible drug inter-actions with your medications, consult your physician or pharmacist.

POSSIBLE SIDE EFFECTS WITH VALPROATE

Common Side Effects

- *Drowsiness and daytime sedation.* The most common complaints with valproate are drowsiness and sedation. If daytime sedation is problematic for the patient, the physician can prescribe the larger dose of Depakote in the evening or at bedtime, or switch to Depakote ER, which can be taken once in the evening or at bedtime.
- *Gastrointestinal (GI) side effects.* The common GI complaints include nausea, vomiting, diarrhea, ab-dominal pain, constipation, and indigestion. GI complaints are more frequent with valproic acid than with the delayed-release or extended-release tablets of Depakote and Depakote ER. Take with food if GI upset occurs.
- *Dizziness and loss of coordination.* These symptoms usually subside as the individual is stabilized on the medication, but if they become intolerable or persist, consult your physician, who may decrease the dose.
- *Tremors.* Patients may experience trembling of fingers and hands, which usually subsides as the they adjust to the medication. If the trembling persists, decreasing the dose may reduce the tremors.
- *Weight gain.* For some individuals, valproate may induce weight gain, especially if it is taken with an antipsychotic medication like olanzapine or lithium. By controlling caloric intake and increasing exer-cise, individuals may control their weight. If weight gain becomes a problem, discuss your concern with your physician.
- *Hair loss (alopecia).* Possible hair loss with valproate may be due to the drug's interference with absorption of zinc and selenium. Some physicians recommend taking vitamins with minerals including zinc and selenium to minimize hair loss while taking valproate.

> **Warning:** Valproate may induce drowsiness and sedation and impair physical coordination and mental alertness. Until you are sure that these side effects will not impair your ability to perform daily tasks, avoid potentially dangerous activities, such as operating a motor vehicle or machinery.

POSSIBLE ADVERSE REACTIONS WITH VALPROATE

- *Liver toxicity* is a rare and unpredictable adverse reaction associated with valproate, which in some cases can lead to fatal liver failure. Young children who are taking valproate for seizures are more vulnerable to liver toxicity than are adults. The risk decreases dramatically with age. In most of the cases reported, liver toxicity was dose-related and reversible when the drug was discontinued. There are no tests to de-termine if an individual is susceptible to liver toxicity from valproate. Liver function tests, however, can help detect early signs of valproate-induced liver abnormalities. In individuals with a history of liver disease, valproate must be used with great caution, if at all. Valproate therapy requires close monitoring of liver function. Blood tests of liver function are recommended before initiation of valproate treatment and should be repeated every 6 months thereafter.

- *Reduced platelets (thrombocytopenia).* Valproate can reduce the number of platelets. Low platelets, or **thrombocytopenia**, may result in delayed blood clotting and potential bleeding. Fortunately, this adverse reaction is rare, but individuals should recognize the early warning signs of thrombocytopenia, including easy bruising, prolonged bleeding time, and frequent nose bleeding.

PREGNANCY AND BREAST FEEDING

The valproates are classified in **Category D** of the FDA Pregnancy Risk Categories. Valproate has been associated with fetal abnormalities when administered during pregnancy. When valproate was administered to pregnant women, especially in the first trimester, it was associated with an increased incidence of neural tube and spinal cord defects (**spina bifida**) in the infant. Valproate should not be administered to pregnant women.

Small amounts of valproate are excreted in breast milk. It is not known what effect valproate may have on the infant if ingested. Women taking valproate should not breastfeed.

If you have any questions about this handout, please consult your physician.

INFORMATION ABOUT

GABAPENTIN (NEURONTIN) AND TOPIRAMATE (TOPAMAX)

FOR PATIENTS AND FAMILIES

Gabapentin (Neurontin) and **topiramate** (Topamax) are anticonvulsants used in the treatment of seizure disorders. However, in psychiatry, they are prescribed for the treatment of mood disorders. Studies suggest gabapentin and topiramate are effective in treating the manic and depressive phases of bipolar disorder. When anticonvulsants such as gabapentin and topiramate are prescribed for mood disorders, they are referred to as *mood stabilizers*.

Anticonvulsants are effective for both seizures and mania because they stabilize "kindling," which consists of unstable, repetitive electrical stimulations of the brain. Once triggered, either by psychological stress or by insult to susceptible areas of the brain, kindling can set off the nervous system, which may result in seizures or manic behavior, depending on how susceptible the individual is.

Gabapentin is available in capsules, tablets, and liquid. The capsules are available in 100-, 300-, and 400-mg strengths, whereas the tablets are available in 600- and 800-mg strengths. In the liquid form, gabapentin is available in a concentration of 250 mg/5 mL. Gabapentin is available only under its brand name **Neurontin** and is not available in generic preparations.

Topiramate is available in tablets and capsules. The tablets come in 25-, 100-, and 200-mg strengths. The capsules are primarily used in pediatric dosing for seizure disorders, as they can be pulled apart and sprinkled in food. Topiramate is available only under its brand **Topamax.**

HOW GABAPENTIN AND TOPIRAMATE ARE PRESCRIBED

The starting dose of gabapentin is usually 300 mg three times a day, and the dosage is increased slowly until clinical response is achieved. The effective dosage for treatment of mood disorders may range from 900 to 2,400 mg/day.

Topiramate is usually initiated at a dosage of 25–50 mg/day, followed by gradual incremental increases of 25 mg per week. Therapeutic dosages for mood stabilization may range from 100 to 300 mg/day.

Monitoring of blood levels for gabapentin and topiramate is unnecessary and is not routinely done.

PROPER USE OF YOUR MEDICATION

Storing Your Medication

- Store your medication in a tamper-resistant vial away from children.
- Store your medication so as to keep it from excessive heat, moisture, and direct light.
- Keep the medication in its original prescription vial with the prescription label intact to prevent others from taking the medication inadvertently.
- Do not use the medication past the expiration date on the label.

Taking Your Medication

- Take your medication exactly as prescribed. Pay close attention to the dosing schedule and do not deviate from your physician's instructions.
- If you miss a dose, take it as soon as possible. However, if it is near the time of your next dose, skip the dose you missed and go back to your regular dosing schedule, but do not double-up the next dose.
- Gabapentin and topiramate may be taken with or without food.
- Since the kidneys are the primary route of elimination for gabapentin and topiramate, maintain adequate fluid intake with your medication, especially with topiramate.

Use of Alcohol and Other Medications

It is recommended that you not consume alcohol while taking gabapentin or topiramate. Alcohol may heighten the drowsiness and sedative effects of these medications.

Antacids should not be taken concomitantly with gabapentin because they may affect the absorption of the medication. If you take an antacid, allow 2 hours before taking gabapentin.

Topiramate is known to decrease the estrogenic component of oral contraceptives (birth-control pills), and the effectiveness of oral contraceptives may be compromised, leading to unintended pregnancy.

When topiramate is used in combination with medications called **carbonic anhydrase inhibitors**, such as **acetazolamide** (Diamox), it may increase the risk of developing kidney stones (see "Possible Adverse Reactions"). The risk of developing kidney stones may be minimized by increasing fluid intake, and hence urinary output, to promote excretion of the drug. If you have any concerns or questions about your medications, consult your physician or pharmacist.

POSSIBLE SIDE EFFECTS

- *Sedation, dizziness, thinking, and memory difficulties.* These side effects of the central nervous system commonly occur with both gabapentin and topiramate and are the most frequently cited reason for discontinuing these medications. Confusion, difficulty with thinking, and memory are frequent complaints from patients taking topiramate at higher dosages. These side effects may be managed by using a larger nighttime dose.
- *Ataxia.* Ataxia is the inability to coordinate movements when walking so that the motion is clumsy, jerky, and uncoordinated. This side effect occurs more commonly with gabapentin. The extent of this problem may be eliminated or minimized by using a larger nighttime dose or by reducing the dosage.
- *Problems with vision.* Occasionally, patients taking gabapentin experience rapid eye movements (nystagmus) and double vision.
- *Fatigue.* This seems to be a common complaint with both gabapentin and topiramate and usually subsides over the course of therapy.
- *Gastrointestinal side effects.* Nausea and loss of appetite are associated with taking topiramate.

Warning: Gabapentin and topiramate may cause sleepiness, dizziness, and other central nervous system side effects. These side effects may be heightened when the medications are used with alcohol. Do not operate a motor vehicle or operate hazardous machinery until you are sure that your medication will not impair your judgment or ability to function.

POSSIBLE ADVERSE REACTIONS

- *Kidney stones*. A small percentage of patients taking topiramate may develop kidney stones. The risk may be higher if the individual also takes **acetazolamide** (Diamox) or a similar type of medication used for treatment of glaucoma (an eye disorder). To minimize the risk of kidney stones, patients taking topiramate are advised to increase fluid intake to promote excretion of the drug.
- *Glaucoma and ocular pain*. In rare cases, topiramate has been associated with glaucoma, an eye disorder marked by increased pressure of the eyeballs and ocular pain. If left untreated, elevated ocular pressure may have serious consequences. Therefore, if you have any visual disturbance or ocular pain, notify your physician immediately.

PREGNANCY AND BREAST FEEDING

Gabapentin and topiramate are classified in **Category C** of the U.S. Food and Drug Administration (FDA) Pregnancy Risk Categories. They are in this category because there are no clinical studies, or there is inadequate information, in women to determine the risks of these agents during pregnancy. Cases of male infants with abnormal development of the penis were reported in pregnant women exposed to topiramate. However, the extent of this risk has not been clearly established with topiramate. In animal studies, at high concentrations, both gabapentin and topiramate demonstrated abnormal fetal developments. Only when benefits outweigh the risks should these medications be prescribed during pregnancy.

Small amounts of gabapentin and topiramate may pass into breast milk. It is not known what effects these drugs have on the infant when ingested. Women taking gabapentin or topiramate should not breastfeed.

If you have questions about this handout, please consult your physician.

INFORMATION ABOUT

LAMOTRIGINE (LAMICTAL)

FOR PATIENTS AND FAMILIES

Lamotrigine (Lamictal) is an anticonvulsant used in the treatment of seizure disorders. However, in psychiatry, it is prescribed for treatment of mood disorders. For bipolar disorder, lamotrigine is effective in treating both manic and depressive episodes. It may also be effective in treating refractory major depression when prescribed in combination with antidepressants. When an anticonvulsant like lamotrigine is prescribed for mood disorders, it is referred to as a *mood stabilizer*. The U.S. Food and Drug Administration (FDA) recently approved lamotrigine for treatment of bipolar disorder.

Anticonvulsants are effective for both seizures and mania because they stabilize "kindling," which consists of unstable, repetitive electrical stimulations of the brain. Once triggered, either by psychological stress or by insult to susceptible areas of the brain, kindling can set off the nervous system, and this may result in seizures or manic behavior, depending on how susceptible the individual is.

Lamotrigine is available in tablets in 25-, 100-, 150-, and 200-mg strengths. Lamictal is not available in a generic form.

HOW LAMOTRIGINE IS PRESCRIBED

Generally, lamotrigine is prescribed when the patient has not fully responded to other mood stabilizers such as **divalproex** (Depakote) and **lithium**. Lamotrigine may be used alone or in combination with lithium or divalproex. The usual starting dose is 25 mg daily for the first week, and then the dosage is increased in 25-mg increments weekly until the desired clinical response is attained. The usual therapeutic dosage range is between 100 and 300 mg/day.

When the patient switches from divalproex to lamotrigine, lamotrigine must be initiated at a lower initial dose until the divalproex is eliminated from the body. If lamotrigine is combined with divalproex, the starting and maintenance doses must be reduced to prevent side effects. Tests to monitor blood levels are usually not required for lamotrigine therapy.

PROPER USE OF YOUR MEDICATION

Storing Your Medication

- Keep your medication in a tamper-resistant vial and out of reach of children.
- Store your medication so as to keep it from excessive heat, moisture, and direct light.
- Keep the medication in it original prescription vial with the prescription label intact to prevent others from taking the medication inadvertently.
- Do not use the medication past the expiration date on the label.

Taking Your Medication

- It is important that you take lamotrigine exactly as prescribed. Pay close attention to the dosing schedule and do not deviate from your physician's instructions.
- If you miss a dose, take it as soon as possible. However, if it is near the time of your next dose, skip the dose you missed and go back to your regular dosing schedule, but do not double-up the next dose.
- Lamotrigine may be taken with food without affecting its absorption.
- Notify your physician immediately if you develop a rash.

Use of Alcohol and Other Medications

It is recommended that you not drink alcohol while taking lamotrigine. Alcohol may alter the metabolism of lamotrigine in the liver and affect its blood levels. Moreover, alcohol may exacerbate the drowsiness and sedation caused by the lamotrigine.

Lamotrigine's metabolism, and hence its levels, may be affected by other drugs. For example, lamotrigine's blood levels may be significantly increased when the drug is administered in combination with **divalproex** (Depakote). On the other hand, **carbamazepine** may decrease the levels of lamotrigine when these drugs are combined. Therefore, it is important that you inform your physician of all the prescription and over-the-counter medications you are taking. If you have questions or concerns, consult your physician or pharmacist.

POSSIBLE SIDE EFFECTS

- *Rash.* Approximately 10% of patients taking lamotrigine develop a localized rash during the first 2–8 weeks of treatment. The incidence of developing rash is even higher when lamotrigine is taken in combination with divalproex. The rash is generalized throughout the body, raised, and red. When the drug is discontinued, the rash eventually disappears. However, in rare cases, the reaction may become more serious and requires immediate medical attention (see "Possible Adverse Reactions"). At the first sign of rash, discontinue lamotrigine and notify your physician immediately. Taking an antihistamine such as **diphenhydramine** (Benadryl) may relieve the itch. **Calamine lotion** may also provide smoothing relief of the burning and itching symptoms.
- *Other common side effects.* Dizziness, sedation, blurred vision and double vision, and difficulty walking (ataxia) can occur.
- *Headaches.*
- *Gastrointestinal side effects.* Nausea, vomiting, and abdominal cramping can occur.

POSSIBLE ADVERSE REACTIONS

- *Life-threatening rashes.* In rare cases, a life-threatening rash, including **Stevens-Johnson syndrome,** is associated with lamotrigine therapy. Stevens-Johnson syndrome is a condition that begins as painful, weeping skin lesions and progresses to organ involvement and failure. It is associated with a high mortality rate. In the majority of cases, life-threatening rashes associated with lamotrigine occurred within 2–8 weeks after initiating therapy. The incidence is higher among younger children; hence, lamotrigine is not recommended for children under 16 years of age, except for patients with certain seizure disorders. Development of rash from lamotrigine is **idiosyncratic;** that is, it is unpredictable and unique to the individual. Since there are no reliable predictors of this adverse reaction, individuals are instructed to monitor for early signs of rash and, when the signs are positive, to discontinue lamotrigine and contact their physician.
- *Hypersensitivity reactions.* In rare cases, life-threatening hypersensitivity reactions to lamotrigine may occur without the development of a rash. The hypersensitivity reaction begins with a fever and swollen lymph nodes and then progresses to organ involvement and failure.

USE IN PREGNANCY AND BREAST FEEDING

Lamotrigine is classified in **Category C** of the U.S. Food and Drug Administration (FDA) Pregnancy Risk Categories. It is given this classification because there are no clinical studies in women, nor is there adequate information, to determine the risk of this agent during pregnancy. However, in studies in rats, lamotrigine decreased concentrations of folic acid (an essential vitamin). Decreased folic acid concentrations during the gestational period are associated with fetal abnormalities. These data imply that lamotrigine, if used during pregnancy, carries some risk to the human fetus as well. Lamotrigine should not be used during pregnancy. Only when the benefits outweigh the risk should lamotrigine be prescribed during pregnancy.

Small amounts of lamotrigine may pass into breast milk and may be ingested by the nursing infant. Since the adverse effects of lamotrigine to the infant are unknown, it is recommended that women not breastfeed.

If you have questions about this handout, please consult your physician.

INFORMATION ABOUT

LITHIUM

FOR PATIENTS AND FAMILIES

Lithium carbonate has been the standard drug therapy for bipolar disorder for over 40 years. When it is prescribed for treatment of mood, such as mania, it is referred to as a *mood stabilizer*. Lithium is effective for controlling acute mania, as well as reducing the frequency of manic and depressive episodes in patients with bipolar disorder.

Lithium also is used to augment antidepressants in treating patients with refractory major depression. Other uses of lithium include treatment of schizophrenic patients with a mood disorder (**schizoaffective disorder**), and treatment of aggression in patients with dementia and mental retardation.

Lithium carbonate is generally dispensed in generic capsules that are available in 150-, 300-, and 600-mg strengths. Lithium carbonate also comes in 300-mg slow-release (**Lithobid**) and 450-mg controlled-release (**Eskalith-CR**) tablets. Delayed-release lithium tablets may be dosed less frequently, and they are less irritating to the stomach than the capsules. Lithium also comes in syrup, **lithium citrate,** in a concentration equivalent to 300 mg of lithium carbonate per 5 mL (1 teaspoonful). For example, 5 mL of lithium citrate is equivalent to a 300-mg capsule of lithium carbonate.

HOW LITHIUM IS PRESCRIBED

In acute mania, higher doses are usually necessary for optimal patient response. Doses vary from 300 to 600 mg three times daily (900–1,800 mg/day) or 450 to 900 mg twice daily with Eskalith-CR tablets. When acute symptoms are stabilized, the dose may be lowered to 300 mg three to four times daily (900–1,200 mg/day). The dose, however, varies from individual to individual. It may take 1–2 weeks for lithium to achieve its full effects.

Antipsychotic medications may be prescribed in conjunction with lithium in acute mania to treat agitation and psychosis until lithium becomes fully effective. The antipsychotic medication may then be gradually decreased and discontinued after the manic episode abates.

Lithium is also used to augment antidepressants in treating refractory depression. When patients fail to respond fully to antidepressants alone, their depression may respond to a combination of an antidepressant and lithium carbonate. This augmentation strategy has been proved effective for treating refractory depression, as well as preventing depressive relapse.

Blood Tests Are Necessary

Blood tests to determine lithium levels are necessary at the beginning of therapy to help the physician determine the therapeutic dose for the patient. At the start of therapy with lithium carbonate, weekly blood levels are obtained, approximately 12 hours after the last dose. Therapeutic levels usually range from 0.6 to 1.2 mEq/L. When the level reaches 1.5 mEq/L or higher, there is concern of toxicity. The dose may need to be lowered, especially when the patient starts to show early signs of lithium toxicity. After the patient is stabilized, and there is no further dosage change, lithium levels may be needed only every 3–6 months, depending on the physician.

Because lithium is eliminated from the body primarily by the kidneys, the patient's renal function must be established before lithium is started. Blood tests for renal function are conducted as part of routine pretreatment tests.

Long-term treatment with lithium may induce hypothyroidism (low function of the thyroid glands). Before lithium therapy is begun, blood tests are ordered to check the patient's thyroid function.

Lithium may interfere with the electrical conduction of the heart. For patients with a history of cardiovascular disease, the physician may order an electrocardiogram (ECG) to check cardiac function and the conduction system to see if there are predisposing risks that may preclude the use of lithium.

PROPER USE OF YOUR MEDICATION

Storage of Your Medication

- Keep your medication in a tamper-resistant vial and out of reach of children. Overdosage of lithium is very dangerous, especially for children.
- Store your medication so as to keep it from excessive heat, moisture, and direct light.
- Keep the medication in it original prescription vial with the prescription label intact to prevent others from taking the medication inadvertently.
- Do not use the medication past the expiration date on the label.
- Do not chew or crush tablets of delayed-release lithium.

Taking Your Medication

- If you miss a dose, take it as soon as possible. However, if it is near the time of your next dose, skip the dose you missed and go back to your regular dosing schedule, but do not double-up the next dose.
- Take lithium with food to avoid stomach upset.
- Drink 8–12 glasses of water or other liquid every day while taking lithium. Maintaining adequate hydration is important for excretion of the drug to prevent toxicity. On hot days, ensure that you maintain adequate fluids to prevent dehydration.
- Recognize symptoms of lithium toxicity and inform your physician when symptoms occur. Early symptoms of lithium toxicity include diarrhea, vomiting, tremor, unsteady balance when standing or walking, drowsiness, and muscular weakness. When these symptoms are present, interrupt your medication and contact your physician.

Use of Alcohol and Other Medications

It is recommended that you not drink alcohol while you are taking lithium. Excessive alcohol intake may result in dehydration and elevation of lithium levels and may increase the risk of lithium toxicity. Furthermore, the depressant effects of alcohol may exacerbate the depressive symptoms of bipolar disorder.

Inform your physicians, including your dentist, that you are taking lithium; medications other doctors prescribe can interact with lithium. For example, thiazide diuretics, such as hydrochlorothiazide, commonly prescribed for high blood pressure, promote sodium excretion, which may enhance lithium retention. Greater amounts of lithium retained by the body may lead to lithium toxicity. Some nonsteroidal anti-inflammatory drugs, including **indomethacin** (Indocin), **ibuprofen** (Motrin), **naproxen** (Aleve, Naprosyn), and **piroxicam** (Feldene), may interfere with the renal excretion of lithium and cause lithium toxicity. If you have questions or concerns, consult your physician or pharmacist.

POSSIBLE SIDE EFFECTS

- *Fine tremors.* With lithium-induced tremors, slight shaking of the fingers is noticeable when the arms are outstretched. Reducing the lithium dosage may treat the tremor. If tremors are severe, it is often a sign that the lithium dose is too high. Notify your physician as soon as possible.
- *Frequent urination.* Lithium may induce frequent urination and excretion of sodium during the early phase of treatment as the body is adjusting to the changes. Maintaining adequate fluids and a normal sodium (salt) diet, especially during the initial stabilization period, is important to prevent enhanced lithium reabsorption and toxicity. It is recommended that patients drink 8–12 glasses of water a day to prevent dehydration.
- *Gastrointestinal (GI) side effects.* GI side effects are frequent complaints. Side effects include nausea, vomiting, abdominal cramping, indigestion, bloated feeling, and excessive salivation. Increasing the dose gradually, taking lithium at mealtime or with snacks, and dividing the doses three to four times a day can minimize these side effects. Using sustained-release tablets may also alleviate GI side effects.
- *Drowsiness and sedation.* A frequent complaint at the start of therapy is drowsiness and sedation, which usually subside as the individual adjusts to the medication. If these symptoms persist, and there is loss of coordination when walking (unstable gait), jerky eye movements, dizziness, confusion, and slurred speech, these may be signs of lithium toxicity. Notify your physician immediately.
- *Weight gain.* Weight gain unrelated to water retention may be a side effect of lithium and may be attributed to increased appetite and caloric intake.
- *Dermatologic (skin) side effects.* Skin rash is reported in about 7% patients taking lithium. Lithium may also exacerbate acne and psoriasis. If these side effects are severe, the physician may be required to lower the lithium dose or switch to another medication.

> **Warning:** Lithium may impair physical coordination and mental alertness needed for performing daily tasks. It is important to avoid potentially dangerous activities, such as operating a motor vehicle, until you are sure that the side effects of lithium will not impair your ability to perform these tasks.

POSSIBLE ADVERSE REACTIONS

- *Hypothyroidism.* As previously discussed, long-term lithium therapy may affect the thyroid glands and diminish thyroid function (**hypothyroidism**). A common laboratory test used to correlate thyroid function is determination of the **thyroid-stimulating hormone** (TSH) level. TSH is a hormone that stimulates the function of the thyroid glands. Elevated levels of TSH, when correlated with positive clinical symptoms, are indicative of hypothyroidism. Clinical signs and symptoms of hypothyroidism may include enlarged thyroid glands, tiredness, intolerance to cold, low energy, and depression. Lithium-induced hypothyroidism may be reversed when the drug is discontinued or when the patient is given supplemental thyroid hormone.
- *Impaired ability of kidneys to concentrate urine.* Infrequently, chronic lithium administration is associated with impairment of the concentrating ability of the kidneys (**nephrogenic diabetes insipidus**). As a result, the individual is unusually thirsty and must drink copious amounts of water, which is lost through frequent urination because the kidneys cannot reabsorb and conserve the body's water. Fortunately, this disorder can be reversed when the lithium dosage is decreased or the lithium is discontinued.
- *Abnormal electrocardiogram (ECG).* Lithium may affect the electrical conduction, and hence the rhythm, of the heart. It may induce changes that show up as an abnormality in an ECG. Although most people taking lithium experience no change in cardiac function, the physician may order a pretreatment ECG for elderly patients or patients who have a history of cardiovascular disease.
- *Lithium toxicity.* There is a narrow margin between therapeutic and toxic levels of lithium. Close monitoring of lithium levels is imperative with lithium administration. Patients should learn to recognize

early symptoms of lithium toxicity, which include drowsiness, diarrhea, vomiting, nausea, muscular weakness, and lack of coordination. At higher lithium levels, toxic symptoms include dizziness, ringing in the ears (**tinnitus**), slurred speech, increasing confusion, blurred vision, inability to coordinate movements (**ataxia**), and twitching of facial muscles and limbs. At very toxic levels, there is a high risk of death from seizures, arrhythmias, and delirium. Thus, early recognition and intervention play an important role in reversing lithium toxicity. When the aforementioned early symptoms develop, the patient should interrupt lithium therapy and contact his or her physician as soon as possible.

PREGNANCY AND BREAST FEEDING

Lithium is classified in **Category D** in the U.S. Food and Drug Administration (FDA) Pregnancy Risk Categories. There is evidence that lithium therapy is associated with human fetal risk during pregnancy. Higher incidences of cardiac and other abnormalities were noted in newborns when women had received lithium during pregnancy. The risk appears to have been greatest when lithium was administered in the first trimester of pregnancy. Therefore, pregnant women should not take lithium, especially during the first trimester of pregnancy. Lithium therapy should only be considered during pregnancy and under very close supervision of the physician when the absolute need for the medication outweighs the potential risk to the fetus.

When women are taking lithium, it is recommended that they not breastfeed, because the drug is excreted into breast milk. When lithium is ingested, it may have harmful effects on the infant's developing nervous system.

If you have any questions about this handout, please consult your physician.

INFORMATION ABOUT

ANTIPARKINSON AGENTS

FOR PATIENTS AND FAMILIES

- Amantadine (Symmetrel)
- Benztropine (Cogentin)
- Biperiden (Akineton)
- Diphenhydramine (Benadryl)
- Procyclidine (Kemadrin)
- Trihexyphenidyl (Artane)

Antiparkinson medications are used primarily in the treatment of **Parkinson's disease**, which is a neurologic disorder that is characterized by tremors, slow movement, a masklike face, rigidity, stooped posture, and drooling. In psychiatry, these agents are used to treat **neuroleptic-induced movement disorders**. Neuroleptics are older antipsychotic medications that induce neurologic side effects that frequently cause movement disorders known as **extrapyramidal syndromes** (EPS). Neuroleptic-induced EPS include parkinsonism, dystonia, and akathisia. Drug-induced **parkinsonism,** as the name implies, has symptoms that mimic primary Parkinson's disease. **Dystonia** is an adverse reaction induced by antipsychotic medications that is manifested by a sudden spasm of the tongue, jaw, neck, and muscles of the eye. Although not an allergic reaction, it can be very frightening for the patient. Dystonias may be treated and rapidly reversed with an injection of benztropine or diphenhydramine. **Akathisia,** another form of EPS, is an inner-driven restlessness caused by antipsychotics. It is described as a feeling of nervousness, with the need to pace and the inability to sit still, muscular discomfort, and agitation.

The antiparkinson medications used for EPS include **anticholinergic agents** (benztropine, biperiden, procyclidine, and trihexyphenidyl); **diphenhydramine**, an antihistamine; and **amantadine**.

How do these medications work? Movement disorder, whether caused by Parkinson's disease or neuroleptic medications, may be exacerbated by excessive activity of the **cholinergic system** because **dopamine**, a neurotransmitter, is diminished in certain areas of the brain. Anticholinergic medications oppose the action of the cholinergic system (i.e., are anticholinergic), facilitating the balance between the cholinergic and dopaminergic systems. Diphenhydramine, although an antihistamine, may work by a similar mechanism because it also possesses anticholinergic activity. **Amantadine,** however, is not an anticholinergic drug and works in ways that are different from anticholinergic agents. Its effect may be achieved by its ability to increase dopamine levels. The advantage of amantadine is that it does not have the side effects of anticholinergic agents, a benefit for the patient who cannot tolerate anticholinergic side effects.

The commonly used antiparkinson medications are listed above by their generic and brand names. Amantadine, benztropine (oral), diphenhydramine, and trihexyphenidyl are available in generic preparations as well. Benztropine (Cogentin) and diphenhydramine (Benadryl) also come in injectable forms for intramuscular administration. Moreover, diphenhydramine has antihistamine activity with a sedative property, and the drug is prescribed commonly for allergies and insomnia.

HOW THESE MEDICATIONS ARE PRESCRIBED

Benztropine is the anticholinergic drug most commonly used for treating neuroleptic-induced parkinsonism and acute dystonia, although other anticholinergics are equally effective. Amantadine is effective for parkinsonism but usually not for acute dystonia. For akathisia, although a trial of an anticholinergic medication or amantadine is reasonable, these agents are generally not effective. A different treatment strategy is usually needed for treating akathisia.

For treatment and prevention of EPS, benztropine (0.5–2 mg two times a day), trihexyphenidyl (2–5 mg three times a day), diphenhydramine (25–50 mg three to four times a day), biperiden (2 mg one to three times a day), procyclidine (5 mg two to three times a day), or amantadine (100–200 mg two times a day) are usually effective. For treatment of an acute dystonic reaction, usually 1–2 mg of benztropine or 50 mg of diphenhydramine, administered in a single intramuscular injection, is effective for aborting the reaction.

Antiparkinson medications are commonly prescribed for prophylaxis (prevention) of EPS with the older, conventional antipsychotics, because these antipsychotics are associated with a high incidence of EPS. The newer, atypical antipsychotics (e.g., olanzapine) have a very low incidence of EPS, and antiparkinson medications may not be needed until EPS occur. The question whether prophylaxis is needed with antipsychotics, and for how long, continues to be debated. Many physicians favor prescribing an anticholinergic agent with conventional antipsychotics, especially with the high-potency agents such as haloperidol. They maintain that prevention of EPS, especially dystonia, is crucial for patients to adhere to their treatment.

PROPER USE OF YOUR MEDICATION

Storing Your Medication

- Keep your medication in a tamper-resistant vial and out of reach of children.
- Store your medication so as to keep it from excessive heat, moisture, and direct light.
- Keep your medication in its original prescription vial with the label intact to prevent others from taking the medication inadvertently.

Taking Your Medication

- Take your medication as instructed by your physician. Do not abruptly stop taking your medication without consulting with your physician. Abrupt discontinuation of anticholinergic agents may result in unpleasant withdrawal symptoms, including irritability, nausea and vomiting, headache, and insomnia. Although anticholinergics are not indicative of addiction, gradual tapering of dosage may be needed before discontinuation of these agents.
- If you miss a dose, take it as soon as possible. However, if it is near the time of your next dose, skip the dose you missed and go back to your regular dosing schedule, but do not double-up the dose.
- You may take your medication with or without food. If the medication upsets your stomach, take it at mealtime.

Use of Alcohol and Other Medications

Patients should refrain from consuming alcohol while taking antiparkinson medications. Some side effects, such as drowsiness and dizziness, may be exacerbated when these medications are combined with alcohol.

Certain medications, including over-the-counter medicines, may interact with the antiparkinson drugs. The drug interaction may *lower* the blood level of the affected drug and decrease the drug's effectiveness; or, it may *elevate* the blood level of the affected drug and cause toxicity. Some medications (e.g., tricyclic antidepressants) have anticholinergic action and may exacerbate the side effects of antiparkinson agents. Inform your physician of all the prescription and over-the-counter medications you are taking. If you have questions about your medications, consult your physician or pharmacist.

POSSIBLE SIDE EFFECTS

In the area of the brain where anticholinergic action is desired, the patient derives therapeutic benefits, but in other areas of the body where such action is undesirable, side effects may occur. Since the cholinergic system is widely distributed throughout the body, anticholinergic agents may interfere with those body functions regulated by the cholinergic system. These side effects are known as **anticholinergic side effects.**

Patients should also be aware that other medications they take may have anticholinergic activity. For example, diphenhydramine (Benadryl), an antihistamine commonly used for allergies and sleep, also has anticholinergic activity.

Possible anticholinergic side effects are as follows:

- Drowsiness and sedation
- Feeling of "spaciness"
- Confusion and memory impairment (especially for the elderly)
- Blurred vision
- Decreased salivation and dry mouth
- Decreased sweating
- Decreased bronchial secretions (exacerbation of asthma and other lung diseases)
- Palpitations
- Constipation
- Delayed or retrograde (flowing backward) ejaculation
- Urinary hesitancy or retention

> **Warning:** These medications may cause drowsiness and dizziness. Exercise caution when engaging in daily activities that require mental alertness, such as operating a motor vehicle. It is recommended that you do not engage in hazardous tasks until you are reasonably certain that your medication does not adversely affect your performance or impair your judgment.

POSSIBLE ADVERSE REACTIONS

- *Seizures.* Amantadine should be used with caution in patients with a history of seizure disorder. Seizures have been reported in patients who were taking amantadine.
- *Heatstroke.* Anticholinergic agents may diminish sweating and compromise the body's ability to dissipate heat. With exposure to hot weather, patients may be susceptible to heatstroke. Elderly patients are especially susceptible. Patients taking large doses of anticholinergic medication and patients taking more than one medication with anticholinergic activity may also be susceptible to heatstroke.
- *Delirium.* Excessive anticholinergic activity, especially from overdosage, may result in a toxic brain reaction known as **delirium**. Delirium is diagnosed by the manifestation of symptoms that include impairment of consciousness with inability to focus or sustain attention, tremors, loss of coordination, restlessness, agitation, and inability to control urination. If left untreated, delirium may be fatal.

    Elderly patients have a higher risk for developing delirium. Other predisposing factors include patients with brain damage, diabetes, alcohol dependence, and malnutrition. In these patients, when a anticholinergic agent is used, lower dosages should be prescribed, especially when the medication is used in combination with other medications with anticholinergic activity.

PREGNANCY AND BREAST FEEDING

Diphenhydramine is classified in **Category B** of the U.S. Food and Drug Administration (FDA) Pregnancy Risk Categories, whereas amantadine, benztropine, biperiden, procyclidine, and trihexyphenidyl are in **Category C.** Diphenhydramine did not show any evidence of fetal risk in animal studies, whereas amantadine, benztropine, biperiden, procyclidine, and trihexyphenidyl showed positive evidence of fetal risk. However, there are no clinical studies with antiparkinson agents in pregnant women, and the data are insufficient, to determine the risk during pregnancy. Antiparkinson agents should be used during pregnancy only if the benefits outweigh the potential risk.

Small amounts of amantadine are excreted in breast milk, but it is not known if the other agents are. Women who take antiparkinson medications should not breastfeed.

If you have any questions about this handout, please consult your physician.

INFORMATION ABOUT

BENZODIAZEPINES

FOR PATIENTS AND FAMILIES

○ **Alprazolam (Xanax)**	○ **Diazepam (Valium)**	○ **Oxazepam (Serax)**
○ **Chlordiazepoxide (Librium)**	○ **Estazolam (ProSom)**	○ **Quazepam (Doral)**
○ **Clorazepate (Tranxene)**	○ **Flurazepam (Dalmane)**	○ **Temazepam (Restoril)**
○ **Clonazepam (Klonopin)**	○ **Lorazepam (Ativan)**	○ **Triazolam (Halcion)**

The **benzodiazepines** are structurally related compounds that have comparable pharmacologic actions. They are used primarily in the treatment of anxiety and insomnia, and benzodiazepines are commonly known as *anti-anxiety* (or *anxiolytic*) and *sedative-hypnotic* agents. A sedative drug reduces nervousness and calms excitement, whereas a hypnotic agent induces drowsiness to facilitate the onset of sleep. Anxiety is an abnormal state of apprehension and fear marked by physical symptoms, including sweating, tension, and palpitations. Anti-anxiety agents, such as benzodiazepines, reduce anxiety and the accompanying physical symptoms. There is essentially no difference between a benzodiazepine that is a sedative and one that is an anxiolytic. Moreover, benzodiazepines in general may be used either as antianxiety or as hypnotic agents, because they act as hypnotics at higher doses and as anxiolytics or sedatives at lower doses.

Benzodiazepines are among the most widely prescribed psychotropic medications. They are proved effective and relatively safe (compared with barbiturates) for the treatment of anxiety disorders and insomnia. In addition, benzodiazepines are used for other psychiatric conditions, including panic disorders, phobias, acute mania, agitation, and alcohol withdrawal. In other areas of medicine, benzodiazepines are used as anticonvulsants, muscle relaxants, and anesthetics. For the purpose of this handout, discussion of benzodiazepines shall focus mainly on antianxiety and sedative-hypnotic agents.

HOW BENZODIAZEPINES ARE PRESCRIBED

The benzodiazepines differ in their potency, duration of action (i.e., half-life), and side effects. They are marketed for use as hypnotics or anxiolytics on the basis of these differences. For example, triazolam (Halcion) has a short duration of action (4–6 hours) and is more suitable for use as a hypnotic agent than diazepam (Valium), which has a much longer duration (over 20 hours). Generally, all the benzodiazepines are equally effective for treating anxiety, and a physician's choice may be based on the medication's different side effects and duration of action. The dosage ranges, half-lives, and common uses of benzodiazepines are summarized in Table 1.

Table 1. Benzodiazepines: Dosage Ranges, Half-Lives, and Common Uses

Drug	Usual dosage range, mg/day[a]	Half-life	Common uses
Alprazolam[b] (Xanax)	1–4	Intermediate	Anxiety disorder, panic disorder, social phobia, posttraumatic stress disorder (PTSD), premenstrual syndrome
Chlordiazepoxide[b] (Librium)	15–100	Intermediate	Anxiety disorders, acute alcohol withdrawal
Clorazepate[b] (Tranxene)	15–60	Long	Anxiety disorder, panic disorders, phobia, acute alcohol withdrawal
Clonazepam[b] (Klonopin)	2–8	Long	Acute mania, agitation, seizure disorders, panic disorder
Diazepam[b] (Valium)	4–40	Very long	Anxiety disorder, panic disorder, PTSD, muscle relaxant, seizure disorder, preoperative anesthesia, alcohol withdrawal
Estazolam (ProSom)	1–2	Short	Sedative-hypnotic
Flurazepam[b] (Dalmane)	15–30	Long	Sedative-hypnotic
Lorazepam[b] (Ativan)	1.5–6	Intermediate	Anxiety disorder, panic disorder, PTSD, phobia, agitation, alcohol withdrawal, premenstrual syndrome
Oxazepam[b] (Serax)	30–120	Intermediate	Anxiety disorder, panic disorder, PTSD, phobia, alcohol withdrawal, premenstrual syndrome
Quazepam (Doral)	7.5–15	Long	Sedative-hypnotic
Temazepam[b] (Restoril)	15–30	Intermediate	Sedative-hypnotic
Triazolam[b] (Halcion)	0.125–0.25	Short	Sedative-hypnotic

[a]Usual dosage ranges for treatment of anxiety or insomnia for the average adult patient.
[b]Generic preparations are available for these benzodiazepines.

PROPER USE OF YOUR MEDICATION

Storing Your Medication

- Keep your medication in a tamper-resistant vial and out of reach of children.
- Store your medication so as to keep it from excessive heat, moisture, and direct light.
- Keep your medication in its original prescription vial with the label intact to prevent someone from inadvertently taking it thinking it is something else.

Taking Your Medication

- Take your medication exactly as instructed by your physician. Do not abruptly stop taking your medication without consulting your physician. Abrupt discontinuation of your medication may result in unpleasant withdrawal symptoms. Benzodiazepines, if taken for any extended period, should be tapered down gradually before terminating the medication completely.
- If you miss a dose, take it as soon as possible. However, if it is near the time of your next dose, skip the dose you missed and go back to your regular dosing schedule, but do not double-up the dose.

Use of Alcohol and Other Medications

Alcohol and other central nervous system (CNS) depressants (e.g., barbiturates, narcotic medications) should not be taken together with benzodiazepines. The interaction of other CNS depressants and benzodiazepines may increase the depressant effects on the brain, producing drowsiness and confusion and impairing coordination. Overdosage of benzodiazepines with CNS depressants is very hazardous. The interaction may result in profound central respiratory depression, decreasing breathing rate and significantly lowering blood pressure. This may result in respiratory and circulatory collapse and can be fatal.

Some medications, including over-the-counter medicines, may interact with benzodiazepines, and they should not be taken together. The drug interaction may *lower* the blood level of the affected drug and decrease the drug's effectiveness; or, it may *elevate* the blood level of the affected drug and cause toxicity. Some medications may decrease the metabolism of certain benzodiazepines and increase their blood levels, resulting in excessive sedation and impairment of coordination. For example, birth-control pills, cimetidine (an anti-ulcer drug), ketoconazole (an antifungal drug), and fluoxetine (an antidepressant), when combined with diazepam, clorazepate, chlordiazepoxide, or alprazolam, may inhibit the metabolism of these benzodiazepines and increase their pharmacologic effects, resulting in excessive sedation, confusion and impaired coordination. Inform your physician of all prescription and over-the-counter medications you are taking. If you have questions about your medications, consult your physician or pharmacist.

POSSIBLE SIDE EFFECTS

- *Drowsiness and sedation.* Daytime sedation and drowsiness are common side effects from benzodiazepines, especially just after taking a dose. In part, excessive sedation may be related to the dose and may be managed by reducing it. Taking the dose close to bedtime may minimize daytime sedation. Usually, patients develop tolerance to the sedative effects of benzodiazepines.

- *Confusion, dizziness, incoordination, and memory impairment.* These side effects may indicate that the dosage is too high for the patient or that the patient may be taking another CNS depressant with the benzodiazepine. Elderly patients are particularly susceptible to these side effects of benzodiazepines, particularly with the longer-acting ones, and are at risk for losing their balance and falling. Reducing the dosage or using a shorter-acting benzodiazepine may mitigate these side effects.

- *Drug dependence.* With prolonged use, benzodiazepines may produce physical dependence and tolerance (i.e., requiring higher doses to achieve the effects previously attained with lower doses). Withdrawal symptoms (see "Possible Adverse Reactions") have occurred in patients after 4–6 weeks of treatment and discontinuation of the benzodiazepine. Individuals with a history of alcohol or substance abuse are at risk for benzodiazepine abuse as well. When benzodiazepines are prescribed and carefully managed under the care of the physician, these medications are very safe.

- *Rebound insomnia.* When a sleeping pill is stopped, patients may experience temporary worsening of sleep disturbance, called **rebound insomnia**. Rebound insomnia is more likely with short-acting hypnotics such as triazolam. Patients may be compelled to continue taking hypnotics, and sometimes taking additional doses, to help them fall back to sleep. Patients should be aware that this effect might lead to overuse of sleeping pills.

Warning: Benzodiazepines may cause drowsiness and dizziness. Exercise caution when engaging in daily activities that require mental alertness, such as operating a motor vehicle. It is recommended that you do not engage in hazardous tasks until you are reasonably certain that your medication does not adversely affect your performance or impair your judgment.

POSSIBLE ADVERSE REACTIONS

- *Withdrawal symptoms.* When benzodiazepines are abruptly discontinued after prolonged treatment, patients may develop withdrawal symptoms. Onset of symptoms may occur in 1–10 days, depending on the half-life of the benzodiazepine. With shorter-acting benzodiazepines (e.g., alprazolam), withdrawal symptoms may occur 2–3 days after ceasing the medication, but with longer-acting ones such as diazepam, symptoms may not emerge until 1–2 weeks later. Withdrawal symptoms from benzodiazepines include anxiety, sweating, nausea, palpitations, fidgeting, jitteriness, poor concentration, and insomnia. Some of these symptoms are due to "rebound" effects from the benzodiazepine (i.e., the original symptoms are made worse upon cessation of the medication).

  The most worrisome reaction from benzodiazepine withdrawal is *seizure.* Fortunately, seizures rarely occur, but patients should be aware of the possibility. When benzodiazepines are being discontinued in patients who have been treated for prolonged periods, the dosages are gradually tapered over 4–8 weeks to avoid withdrawal symptoms, especially in patients with a history of seizures. Therefore, patients should not abruptly discontinue their benzodiazepine without first consulting with their physician.

- *Paradoxical reactions.* Similar to the effects of alcohol in some patients, benzodiazepines may paradoxically precipitate excitation, stimulation, and loss of inhibition (disinhibition), which may lead to anxiety, aggressive behavior, anger, rage, and violence. Patients who may be susceptible to these reactions include the elderly, individuals with brain damage, and individuals with a history of aggressive, antisocial behavior

- *Amnesia.* Reports of amnesia in patients taking triazolam (Halcion) have raised concerns with this benzodiazepine. It was a hypnotic favored by travelers for inducing sleep during long flights, because triazolam is short-acting and does not have the "hangover" effects of longer-acting hypnotics. After taking triazolam, these patients could not recall what they did the next day, although they went about their usual business. Amnesia has also been reported with other benzodiazepines, but data suggest there is a higher incidence of amnesia with triazolam, particularly with the 0.5-mg dose. It is recommended that patients not exceed a 0.25-mg dose of triazolam, and they should not consume alcohol after taking it.

PREGNANCY AND BREAST FEEDING

The benzodiazepines and their metabolites (the byproducts of metabolism) are known to freely cross the placenta, and they pose a risk to the developing fetus, especially during the first trimester of pregnancy. Use of benzodiazepines during pregnancy is associated with development of cleft lip or palate and congenital heart problems. Hence, benzodiazepines fall into **Category D** or **X** of the U.S. Food and Drug Administration (FDA) Pregnancy Risk Categories. Benzodiazepines in Category D include alprazolam, chlordiazepoxide, clonazepam, clorazepate, diazepam, lorazepam, and oxazepam; those in Category X include estazolam, temazepam, and triazolam. Drugs in Category D show positive evidence of human fetal risk, and they should be avoided during pregnancy. However, a drug in this risk group is not absolutely contraindicated for use during pregnancy, especially if it is needed in a life-threatening situation because safer drugs are ineffective. Drugs in Category X are **contraindicated** for use during pregnancy because they have demonstrated fetal abnormalities in animal or human studies.

Moreover, benzodiazepines may reach fetal circulation and accumulate in the fetus. Newborns who have been exposed to benzodiazepines show signs of withdrawal symptoms, including irritability, tremors, and respiratory problems.

Benzodiazepines are excreted in breast milk. Women who are taking a benzodiazepine should not breastfeed. There may be harmful effects to the infant's developing nervous system if the infant absorbs the drug.

If you have any questions about this handout, please consult your physician.

INFORMATION ABOUT

BUSPIRONE (BUSPAR)

FOR PATIENTS AND FAMILIES

Buspirone (BuSpar) is used in the treatment of anxiety disorders. It is unlike the benzodiazepines or Valium-like medications, which are widely used for treatment of anxiety. Buspirone is used to treat generalized anxiety disorder, anxiety with associated depressive symptoms, and social anxiety disorder. It may benefit people who have both depression and anxiety. Generally, buspirone is not effective in treating panic disorder, but it may be useful in treating obsessive-compulsive disorder (OCD) and aggression.

Buspirone produces less sedation than the benzodiazepine medications. Unlike the benzodiazepines, it does not induce physical or psychological dependence.

Buspirone comes in tablets in 5-, 10-, and 15-mg strengths. It is marketed under the brand **BuSpar** but is also available generically.

HOW BUSPIRONE IS PRESCRIBED

The usual starting dose is 5 mg two or three times a day. The dose is then gradually increased as needed to alleviate symptoms of anxiety. This slow approach minimizes possible side effects. Doses vary from patient to patient and for different conditions. By the second week, the dose of buspirone is usually increased to 10 mg two to three times a day. The usual maintenance dosage is 20–30 mg/day; the maximum daily dose should not exceed 60 mg.

Depending on the nature of the anxiety disorder or symptoms, buspirone may be needed for a short period or for many years. For example, if anxiety is a symptom of some other psychiatric condition, buspirone may be needed only until symptoms abate. In treating generalized anxiety disorder, however, buspirone may be needed much longer to suppress symptoms. When buspirone has been successful in treating anxiety, it usually continues to suppress symptoms for as long as it is administered. When there is a need to discontinue buspirone, the process should be done gradually by tapering the dose before discontinuation.

PROPER USE OF YOUR MEDICATION

Storing Your Medication

- Keep your medication in a tamper-resistant vial and out of reach of children.
- Store your medication so as to keep it from excessive heat, moisture, and direct light.
- Keep your medication in its original prescription vial with the label intact to prevent others from taking the medication inadvertently.
- Do not use your medication past the expiration date found on the prescription label.

Taking Your Medication

- If you miss a dose, take it as soon as possible. However, if it is near the time of your next dose, skip the dose you missed and go back to your regular dosing schedule, but do not double-up on the dose.

- The full anti-anxiety effects of buspirone may take 2–4 weeks. If you stop your medication before then, you may think the medication is ineffective.

Use of Alcohol and Other Medications

It is recommended that you do not drink alcohol while taking buspirone. The sedative effects of buspirone may worsen with alcohol. Drinking excessive alcohol may also exacerbate anxiety and depression. Some medications, including over-the-counter medicines, may interact with buspirone. The drug interaction may *lower* the blood level of the affected drug and decrease the drug's effectiveness; or, it may *elevate* the blood level of the affected drug and cause toxicity.

Monoamine oxidase inhibitors (MAOIs), a class of antidepressants that includes **phenelzine** (Nardil) and **tranylcypromine** (Parnate), should not be taken with buspirone. The combination may dangerously elevate blood pressure. Inform your physician of all the prescription and over-the-counter medications you are taking. If you have any questions or concerns with your medications, consult your physician or pharmacist.

POSSIBLE SIDE EFFECTS

Generally, buspirone is well tolerated and has few serious side effects. Commonly, side effects occur shortly after starting therapy and when the dose is increased. Common side effects include the following:

- *Drowsiness.* Buspirone is less sedating than the other benzodiazepines, but patients may experience some sedating effects from the medication.
- *Nervousness.* Paradoxically, in the clinical trials, some patients complained of nervousness from this medication for treatment of anxiety.
- *Headaches.*
- *Nausea.*
- *Insomnia.*

Warning: Buspirone may induce dizziness, light-headedness, or drowsiness for some people, which may impair physical coordination and mental alertness for performing daily tasks. It is important to avoid potentially dangerous activities, such as driving a car, until you are sure that the side effects of buspirone will not put you or someone else in danger.

USE IN PREGNANCY AND BREAST FEEDING

Buspirone is classified in **Category B** of the U.S. Food and Drug Administration (FDA) Pregnancy Risk Categories. It has not been studied in women, so no conclusions can be drawn regarding the safety of its use during pregnancy. Animal studies have not shown buspirone to cause fetal abnormalities. Buspirone should be taken during pregnancy only when the need for the medication outweighs the potential risk to the fetus.

The extent of excretion in breast milk of buspirone is unknown. It is recommended that women taking buspirone not breastfeed.

If you have any questions about this handout, please consult your physician.

INFORMATION ABOUT

ZALEPLON (SONATA) AND ZOLPIDEM (AMBIEN)

FOR PATIENTS AND FAMILIES

Hypnotic medications are used for treatment of insomnia, which is the inability to fall asleep or maintain adequate sleep. Insomnia may be due to a primary sleep disorder or a part of a wider symptom profile of other psychiatric disorders (e.g., anxiety) or medical condition (e.g., pain). Medications can sometimes cause insomnia. For example, the antidepressants known as **selective serotonin reuptake inhibitors** (SSRIs), such as **fluoxetine** (Prozac), may induce insomnia. **Caffeine** is also well known for its effect on sleep disturbance.

Zaleplon (Sonata) and **zolpidem** (Ambien) are **nonbenzodiazepine** (benzodiazepines include diazepam *[Valium]* and *Valium-like* medications) **hypnotics** used for treating insomnia. They induce and maintain sleep without affecting normal sleep stages. Zaleplon, zolpidem, and the newer, short-acting benzodiazepines have generally replaced older hypnotics such as the barbiturates and chloral hydrate.

Zolpidem has a duration of action of 6–8 hours. It helps to induce sleep and maintains normal sleep stages without increasing daytime drowsiness as do benzodiazepine hypnotics, such as temazepam (Restoril). Zaleplon is a very-short-acting hypnotic, with a half-life of about 1 hour. Zaleplon is helpful for those who have difficulty falling asleep or those who wake up at night and have difficulty falling back to sleep. Like zolpidem, zaleplon maintains normal sleep stages.

Both zolpidem and zaleplon cause minimal rebound insomnia (i.e., temporary worsening of insomnia soon after discontinuation of the hypnotic) and withdrawal symptoms (i.e., development of side effects upon abrupt discontinuation of the hypnotic) as compared with benzodiazepines, and they have less potential for addiction and abuse than the barbiturates and benzodiazepines. Moreover, zaleplon and zolpidem may continue to be effective for up to 6 months, whereas benzodiazepine hypnotics like triazolam lose their efficacy after 2 weeks of treatment.

Both zaleplon and zolpidem are available in tablets in 5- and 10-mg strengths and are marketed under their brand without any generic competition.

HOW ZALEPLON AND ZOLPIDEM ARE PRESCRIBED

The dose for zaleplon and zolpidem is a 10-mg tablet shortly before bedtime. Elderly patients and debilitated patients may need a dose of only 5 mg. The dose for zaleplon and zolpidem should not exceed 10 mg.

PROPER USE OF YOUR MEDICATION

Storing Your Medication

- Keep your medication in a tamper-resistant vial and out of reach of children.
- Store your medication so as to keep it from excessive heat, moisture, and direct light.
- Keep your medication in its original prescription vial with the label intact to prevent someone from inadvertently taking it thinking it is something else.

Taking Your Medication

- Take your medication exactly as instructed by your physician. Do not take more than the dose prescribed.
- Zaleplon and zolpidem have a rapid onset of action and should only be taken immediately prior to going to bed or during the night when there is difficulty falling asleep. Allow at least 4–6 hours of sleep before resuming daily activities.

Use of Alcohol and Other Medications

Zaleplon and zolpidem are central nervous system (CNS) depressants that should not be taken with alcohol or other CNS depressants (e.g., barbiturates, benzodiazepines, narcotic medications). They should only be taken shortly before going to bed when needed for sleep. If alcohol or a CNS-depressant medication was consumed prior to bedtime, do not take the sleep medication. Wait at least several hours to see if it is needed.

Some medications, including over-the-counter medicines, may adversely interact with zaleplon or zolpidem, and they should not be taken concomitantly. The drug interaction may *lower* the blood level of the affected drug and decrease the drug's effectiveness; or, it may *elevate* the blood level of the affected drug and cause toxicity. Other depressants may increase zaleplon and zolpidem's effects, resulting in excessive sedation, confusion, and impairment of coordination. Inform your doctor of all prescription and over-the-counter medications you are taking. If you have questions about your medications, consult your physician or pharmacist.

Duration of Therapy

If possible, hypnotics should be used for the short-term treatment of insomnia, generally requiring no more than 1–2 weeks of treatment. If the patient's sleep disturbance is a wider symptom of a medical illness or psychiatric disorder, treatment of that condition should be the primary goal. Some patients may require longer than the recommended use of a hypnotic, but each case must be carefully evaluated and monitored to prevent a developing dependency from chronic use.

In general, patients develop tolerance to hypnotics over the course of several weeks of continuous treatment. Hypnotics become less effective for insomnia over time, and a larger dose may be needed to deliver the same hypnotic effect. With zaleplon and zolpidem, there is very little evidence of this side effect, and these hypnotics may continue to be effective for 4–5 weeks, and perhaps for as long as 6 months.

POSSIBLE SIDE EFFECTS

- *Daytime drowsiness and fatigue.* Daytime drowsiness and fatigue are infrequent with zaleplon or zolpidem. Their occurrence may indicate too large of a dose for the patient, especially for elderly patients. Drowsiness and fatigue can be managed by reducing the bedtime dose.
- *Confusion, dizziness, loss of coordination, and memory impairment.* Zaleplon and zolpidem may produce additive depressant effects when taken with other CNS depressants, including alcohol, narcotic medications, and benzodiazepines. Excessive CNS-depressant effects may result in confusion, dizziness, loss of coordination, and impairment of memory. Elderly patients may be particularly susceptible to these side effects. Dosage reduction may be needed when zaleplon and zolpidem are coadministered with other CNS-depressant medications.
- *Drug dependence and abuse.* With regular and chronic use of zaleplon and zolpidem, there is a risk of dependence. Withdrawal symptoms (see "Possible Adverse Reactions") have occurred in patients after long-term use of these agents when discontinued. Individuals with a history of alcohol or substance abuse may be predisposed to a greater risk of dependency and abuse of zaleplon and zolpidem. However, when zaleplon and zolpidem are prescribed and carefully monitored under the care of the physician, these medications are very safe.

> **Warning**: Zaleplon and zolpidem may cause drowsiness and sedation. They should be used at bedtime when you expect to get 4–6 hours of sleep before engaging in daily activities. Exercise caution when engaging in daily activities that require mental alertness, such as operating a motor vehicle, until you are reasonably certain that your medication does not adversely affect your performance or impair your judgment.

POSSIBLE ADVERSE REACTIONS

- *Withdrawal symptoms.* When zaleplon and zolpidem are abruptly discontinued after daily use for an extended period of time, patients may develop withdrawal symptoms. Withdrawal symptoms include anxiety, sweating, nausea, palpitations, fidgeting, jitteriness, poor concentration, and insomnia. Some of these symptoms may be due to "rebound" effects from the medication (i.e., the original symptoms are made worse upon cessation of the sleep medication).
- *Paradoxical reactions.* Similar to the effects of alcohol and benzodiazepines in some patients, zaleplon and zolpidem may precipitate a paradoxical reaction of excitation, stimulation, and loss of inhibition (disinhibition). This reaction may lead to aggressive behavior, agitation, or behavior that seems out of character for the individual. Patients who are susceptible to these reactions include the elderly, individuals with brain damage, and individuals with a history of aggressive or antisocial behavior.
- *Memory problems.* There have been reports of amnesia in patients taking zaleplon and zolpidem. Generally, the patient may not remember what happened for several hours after taking the sleep medication. This type of amnesia was reported when zaleplon or zolpidem was taken while traveling, especially during airflight, and the individual woke up before the effect of the medication wore off. By allowing 7–8 hours of sleep after taking zaleplon or zolpidem, memory problems are usually avoided.

PREGNANCY AND BREAST FEEDING

Zolpidem and zaleplon are classified in **Categories B** and **C** of the U.S. Food and Drug Administration (FDA) Pregnancy Risk Categories, respectively. Zolpidem is in Category B because there is no evidence of risk in humans. There are no adequate studies of zolpidem in pregnant women. However, animal studies showed some adverse maternal and fetal effects from zolpidem. Zaleplon was placed in Category C because risk in humans cannot be ruled out. There are no adequate studies of zaleplon in pregnant women to guide clinicians in determining the risk in humans; however, animal studies have demonstrated positive fetal risk in rats. It is recommended that women not use sedative-hypnotics during pregnancy. At birth, babies exposed to sedative-hypnotics during pregnancy showed signs of withdrawal symptoms, including irritability, tremors, and respiratory problems.

Both zaleplon and zolpidem are excreted in small amounts in breast milk. Women who are taking these sleep medications should not breastfeed. It is unknown whether there are harmful effects to the nursing infant when ingested.

If you have any questions about this handout, please consult your physician.

INFORMATION ABOUT

NONSTIMULANTS FOR THE TREATMENT OF ATTENTION-DEFICIT/HYPERACTIVITY DISORDER

FOR PATIENTS AND FAMILIES

○ **Atomoxetine (Strattera)**

○ **Clonidine (Catapres, Catapres-TTS)**

○ **Guanfacine (Tenex)**

Atomoxetine (Strattera), **clonidine** (Catapres), and **guanfacine** (Tenex) are medications used in the treatment of attention-deficit/hyperactivity disorder (ADHD). These agents are chemically unrelated to stimulants, such as the amphetamines and methylphenidate, and work in ways different than do stimulants to enhance cognitive function and decrease hyperactivity in children with ADHD. The U.S. Food and Drug Administration (FDA) approved atomoxetine for the treatment of ADHD, while clonidine and guanfacine are approved for the treatment of high blood pressure (hypertension), but not for ADHD. Clonidine and guanfacine are used *off-label* when prescribed for nonapproved indications. The FDA restricts pharmaceutical companies to marketing and advertising their drug products for approved indications only. This restriction, however, does not limit physicians from prescribing drugs for nonapproved indications when scientific data and clinical experience support their use for other treatments. Although clonidine and guanfacine are commonly known as antihypertensive medications, they are used in psychiatry for treating ADHD and other disorders.

Clonidine and guanfacine have also proved effective in the treatment of tic disorders, including Tourette's syndrome. A *tic* is a sudden movement, gesture, or verbal outburst that can range from a simple movement such as as eye blinking or head jerk to a more complex facial expression or gesture of the arms or head. Tics are manifested as phonic or vocal tics, which range from throat-clearing sounds to utterance of words or speech that often are obscene. Some patients have a diagnosis of ADHD and a tic disorder, and clonidine and guanfacine are very effective for treatment in these cases.

Atomoxetine, clonidine, and guanfacine have a common action: these agents enhance the transmission of **norepinephrine**, a neurotransmitter in the brain. Studies of patients with ADHD suggest that an abnormal function of the norepinephrine system may in part be responsible for the inattentive and hyperactive problems seen with the disorder. By increasing the level of norepinephrine, these agents may reduce the symptoms of ADHD, and this could account for the positive results seen in treated children.

Unlike amphetamines and methylphenidate, atomoxetine, clonidine, and quanfacine have a much lower potential for abuse. These agents do not provide the reinforcing, euphoric effects that lead to addiction as do stimulants. They are prescription medicines but are not classified as controlled substances.

Atomoxetine, a recently introduced medicine for use in treating ADHD, comes in 10-, 18-, 25-, 40-, and 60-mg capsules and is available only under the brand **Strattera**. Clonidine comes in 0.1-, 0.2-, and 0.3-mg tablets. It is also available in topical patches, which need to be changed only once a week. Clonidine tablets are available in generic preparations, but the topical patches are available only under the brand **Catapres**. Guanfacine comes in 1- and 2-mg tablets and is available in generic preparations.

HOW THESE MEDICATIONS ARE PRESCRIBED

Atomoxetine is indicated for treatment of ADHD in children over 6 years of age and adults. The starting dose for smaller children who weigh less than 50 pounds is calculated on the basis of the body weight. For children over 50 pounds, adolescents, and adults, the starting dose is 40 mg, which may be administered as a single dose in the morning or in evenly divided doses in the morning and afternoon. The dose may be increased no sooner than 3 days to a total daily dose of 80 mg, administered once or twice a day. After 2–4 more weeks, the dose may be increased, if needed, to a maximum total daily dose of 100 mg. Atomoxetine may be taken with or without food.

Clonidine and guanfacine may be prescribed alone (monotherapy) or in combination with a stimulant in the treatment of ADHD. Unlike stimulants, which may cause insomnia, clonidine and guanfacine are sedating and are sometimes prescribed in the evening to offset insomnia that may result from an earlier dose of stimulant.

The pediatric doses for clonidine and guanfacine are based on body weight. The standard dosage ranges for ADHD are 0.1 to 0.3 mg/day for clonidine and 0.5 to 4 mg/day for guanfacine. To prevent daytime sedation, most physicians start clonidine and guanfacine with only a bedtime dose. As the dosage is increased, clonidine and guanfacine are administered in divided doses. Clonidine, with a shorter duration of action than guanfacine, is usually administered two to four times daily, whereas guanfacine is administered two to three times daily.

Clonidine patches (Catapres-TTS) come in the same strengths as the tablets (i.e., 0.1, 0.2, and 0.3 mg). For treatment of ADHD, clonidine patches may have to be changed every 5 days rather than every 7 days, as stated by the manufacturer for controlling high blood pressure.

PROPER USE OF YOUR MEDICATION

Storing Your Medication

- Keep the medication in a tamper-resistant vial and out of reach of children. Clonidine topical patches should be kept in their foil packets unopened until ready for use.
- Store the medication so as to keep it from excessive heat, moisture, and direct light.
- Keep the medication in its original prescription vial with the label intact to prevent someone from inadvertently taking the medication.

Taking Your Medication

- Take the medication exactly as instructed by the physician. Do not abruptly stop taking clonidine or guanfacine because it may result in unpleasant side effects (see "Possible Adverse Reactions"). Clonidine and guanfacine should be gradually reduced over several days to avoid a reaction.
- If you missed a dose, take it as soon as possible, but if it near the time of the next dose, skip the dose you missed and go back to the regular dosing schedule. Do not double-up on the dose.
- Apply the clonidine patch to a clean, dry, and hairless area of the skin on the upper arm or back. If the patch comes off, apply an adhesive overlay directly over the patch. Use a different skin site from the previous application.

Use of Alcohol and Other Medications

Patients (adults and teenagers) should not consume alcohol, since it may exacerbate the symptoms of ADHD. The depressant effects of alcohol may be made worse by clonidine and guanfacine. Some medications, including over-the-counter medicines, may interact with atomoxetine, clonidine, or guanfacine, and they should not be taken concomitantly. The drug interaction may *lower* the blood level of the affected drug and decrease the drug's effectiveness; or, it may *elevate* the blood level of the affected drug and cause toxicity. Atomoxetine should not be taken with antidepressants known as **monoamine oxidase inhibitors** (MAOIs) or within 2 weeks after stopping an MAOI. The combination may result in a severe adverse reaction (see "Possibe Adverse Effects").

POSSIBLE SIDE EFFECTS

Side effects reported with clonidine and guanfacine include

- Dry mouth
- Drowsiness and sedation
- Dizziness
- Headaches
- Nightmares and frequent waking at night
- Nausea and vomiting
- Weight gain
- Lowered blood pressure (hypotension) and slow heart rate

Side effects reported with atomoxetine include

- Headaches
- Sedation
- Dizziness
- Nausea and vomiting
- Abdominal pain
- Constipation
- Loss of appetite
- Elevated blood pressure and heart rate

POSSIBLE ADVERSE REACTIONS

- *Rebound reaction.* Abrupt discontinuation of clonidine or guanfacine (but less frequently) may result in a rebound reaction, consisting of elevated blood pressure, nervousness, agitation, and headache.
- *Cardiovascular effects.* Clonidine and guanfacine are medications used primarily for lowering blood pressure (antihypertensive medications). They must be used with caution in patients with a history of heart disease. In patients with a history of heart block, these agents should not be used, as they may dangerously slow the heart rate. Blood pressure and pulse should be monitored routinely during treatment with clonidine and guanfacine. Atomoxetine has been reported to *elevate* blood pressure and heart rate and should be used with caution in patients with high blood pressure.
- *Depression.* Clonidine has been reported to exacerbate or precipitate depression in some children.
- *Drug interaction with atomoxetine.* An MAOI antidepressant should not be taken concomitantly with atomoxetine. The combination of the two drugs can precipitate a marked elevation of blood pressure **(hypertensive crisis)**.
- *Growth suppression.* Growth suppression has been reported in children treated with atomoxetine. However, the extent of growth suppression may not be as clinically significant as with stimulants. It is recommended that routine measurements of height and weight be taken during treatment with atomoxetine.

PREGNANCY AND BREAST FEEDING

Atomoxetine and clonidine are classified in **Category C** of the U.S. Food and Drug Administration (FDA) Pregnancy Risk Categories. Atomoxetine and clonidine are in this category because they have been shown to produce fetal abnormalities in animals. However, clinical studies are lacking to determine their fetal risk in humans.

Guanfacine is classified in **Category B**; it was placed in this category because it was not shown to produce fetal abnormalities in animals. Its risks in humans, however, cannot be concluded because there are no controlled studies, or there are inadequate data, to determine fetal risk.

Atomoxetine, clonidine, and guanfacine are excreted in breast milk. It is recommended that the mother not breastfeed if these medications are needed.

If you have any questions about this handout, please consult your physician.

INFORMATION ABOUT

AMPHETAMINES AND METHYLPHENIDATE

FOR PATIENTS AND FAMILIES

○ **Dextroamphetamine (Dexedrine, Dexedrine Spansules)**

○ **Amphetamine Mixtures (Adderall, Adderall XR)**

○ **Methylphenidate (Ritalin, Ritalin-SR, Metadate ER, Metadate-CD, Concerta)**

The medications in this group are known as **psychostimulants**, or are simply referred to as stimulants. These agents are used primarily for the treatment of **attention-deficit/hyperactivity disorder** (ADHD). With over six decades of clinical experience and numerous clinical studies, stimulants have been shown to improve outcome in children with ADHD. Stimulants increase their ability to concentrate, extend attention span, and decrease hyperactivity and impulsivity, and oppositional behavior. Similarly, in the treatment of adults, who frequently have a history of childhood ADHD, stimulants help the individuals concentrate and remain focused on their tasks, increase their attention span, and decrease impulsivity and hyperactivity.

The cause of ADHD is unknown, but the clinical evidence implicates the dopamine and norepinephrine neuropathways in different areas of the brain. Dopamine and norepinephrine are neurotransmitters (i.e., brain chemicals that facilitate communication between brain cells) that have been studied and shown to be involved in attention, concentration, motivation, interest, and learning. Stimulants such as amphetamine and methylphenidate enhance levels of these neurotransmitters in the brain. It may seem paradoxical that stimulants have a calming effect—namely, they decrease hyperactivity and increase mental focusing—in ADHD, when the opposite effect from these agents would be expected. Because ADHD may be due to a "biochemical imbalance" of dopamine and norepinephrine in the areas of the brain that affect concentration, attentiveness, and impulse control, stimulants work by increasing levels of these neurotransmitters and resetting the biochemical balance to diminish the symptoms of ADHD.

CONCERNS WITH USE OF PSYCHOSTIMULANTS

The most common concern with the long-term use of stimulants for treating ADHD is dependence and abuse of these substances. Stimulants are tightly regulated prescription medications because they have a high potential for abuse. However, stimulants are very safe when prescribed and monitored under the care of a physician. Long-term studies have shown that children treated with these agents are not at greater risk for abusing stimulants than are other children. Contrary to opinion, compelling evidence showed that aggressive treatment of ADHD with psychostimulants during childhood resulted in better outcome as teenagers and adults. As a result, these children did better in school and attained higher educational levels than children who did not receive stimulants; they showed less aggression, and they had fewer automobile accidents and problems with alcohol and drug abuse as teenagers.

Another common concern with use of stimulants in children is that these agents may suppress growth. During treatment with stimulants, children may experience suppression of their growth. However, generally the suppression is temporary, and children regain their height. Physicians usually provide drug-free holidays in the summers or weekends, when the medication may not be needed as much as during school time, to allow children's growth to catch up. Follow-up studies of stimulant-treated children into adulthood showed no significant impairment in their height.

HOW THESE MEDICATIONS ARE PRESCRIBED

Methylphenidate is the most widely prescribed stimulant for ADHD, but dextroamphetamine is equally effective. If one stimulant is not effective, the patient may respond to the other agent. Immediate-release methylphenidate is short acting and begins to work 30–60 minutes after administration, with a duration of 2–5 hours. The advantage is that this form works quickly, but the duration of medication is short and frequently requires dosing two to three times a day. Usually, methylphenidate is administered in divided doses in the morning and at noon (e.g., before school and before lunchtime). By evening, methylphenidate wears off and is most likely not to interfere with sleep at bedtime.

However, some children may require a third dose around 4 P.M. when methylphenidate wears off and hyperactive behavior may be unmanageable in the evening.

Like methylphenidate, immediate-release dextroamphetamine is a short-acting stimulant. Peak effects are seen 1–2 hours after administration, and the effects of the medication last 2–5 hours. The usual dosing with dextroamphetamine is two to three times daily.

Since multiple dosing may be difficult for children during days at school, physicians may prescribe a long-acting methylphenidate or dextroamphetamine, which can provide 8–12 hours of benefit from a single morning dose. The different designations of the long-acting stimulants are confusing—for example, Ritalin-SR, "*SR*" for *sustained-release*; Ritalin-LA, "*LA*" for *long acting*; Metadate ER, "*ER*" for *extended-release*; Metadate-CD, "*CD*" for *controlled-delivery*; Adderall XR, "*XR*" for *extended-release*; and Dexedrine *Spansule,* a trademark for a *long-acting* capsule form.

A mixture of dextroamphetamine and amphetamine is available under the brand name **Adderall**, which comes in immediate- and extended-release forms. The immediate-release preparation of Adderall provides duration of action for about 5 hours, whereas the extended-release form, **Adderall XR**, is effective most of day with a single morning dose. The stimulants, their dosage forms, and usual dosage ranges are summarized in Table 1.

Dosing of stimulants is individualized on the basis of age, weight, and clinical presentation of symptoms. For example, the usual starting dose of dextroamphetamine for children between the ages of 3 and 5 years is 2.5 mg once a day given in the mornings; the dosage is increased in increments of 2.5 mg/day at weekly intervals until adequate response is attained. For children 6 years and older, the usual starting dose is 5 mg once or twice a day, and the dosage is increased in increments of 5 mg/day at weekly intervals. The maximum dosage for dextroamphetamine in all age groups should not exceed 40 mg/day. Once the daily dose is established, the patient may be switched to a longer-acting agent (Dexedrine Spansules or Adderall XR) for the convenience of once-a-day administration.

For children 6 years and older, the usual starting dose of immediate-release methylphenidate is 5 mg before breakfast and lunch, and the dose is increased by 5–10 mg in weekly intervals as needed. The maximum dosage for methylphenidate should not exceed 60 mg/day. Patients may be converted from the immediate-release methylphenidate to a single dose of the long-acting preparation. For example, if the patient was taking a 10-mg tablet of regular methylphenidate in the morning and afternoon, the medication could be switched to a single dose of a 20-mg sustained-release tablet (e.g., Ritalin-SR), which has a duration of approximately 8 hours. If control is needed for longer than 8 hours, one of the extended-release preparations (e.g., Ritalin-LA, Metadate-CD, or Concerta) may be substituted. For example, if the patient was taking 5 mg methylphenidate three times a day, switching to a single 18-mg capsule of Concerta in the morning could provide control for 10–12 hours.

Table 1. Stimulants Commonly Used for the Treatment of ADHD

Generic name	Trade name	Available strengths	Dosing frequency
Dextroamphetamine Immediate-release	Dexedrine	5, 10 mg (tablets)	One or two times a day
Dextroamphetamine Sustained-release	Dexedrine Spansules	5, 10, 15 mg (capsules)	Once a day in the morning
Amphetamine/ dextroamphetamine mixture	Adderall	5, 7.5, 10, 12.5, 15, 20, 30 mg (tablets)	Two or three times a day
	Adderall XR	5, 10, 15, 20, 25, 30 mg (capsules)	Once a day in the morning
Methylphenidate	Ritalin	5, 10, 20 mg (tablets)	Two to three times a day
Sustained-release	Ritalin-SR	20 mg (tablet)	Once a day in the morning
Extended-release	Metadate ER	10, 20 mg (tablets)	Once a day in the morning
Long-acting	Ritalin-LA	20, 30, 40 mg (capsules)	Once a day in the morning
Controlled-delivery	Metadate-CD	20 mg (capsule)	Once a day in the morning
Extended-release	Concerta	18, 27, 36, 54 mg (capsules)	Once a day in the morning

With recent advances in drug delivery systems, manufacturers have incorporated these new technologies in stimulants that provide both an immediate action and an extended action of the drug in a single capsule. For example, Concerta uses a drug delivery system that releases 22% methylphenidate within the first hour and the remainder of the drug over the next 10 hours. The system delivers a slow and steady absorption of the drug into the body without the peaks and valleys of the immediate-release preparations. Extended-release stimulants using these new drug delivery systems may be associated with fewer, and less intense, side effects when compared with the older agents. Physicians are more likely to have patients who are new to stimulant treatment begin taking a long-acting preparation.

PROPER USE OF YOUR MEDICATION

Storing Your Medication

- Keep the medication in a tamper-resistant vial and out of reach of children.
- Store the medication so as to keep it from excessive heat, moisture, and direct light.
- Keep the medication in its original prescription vial with the label intact to prevent someone from inadvertently taking the medication.

Taking Your Medication

- Take the medication exactly as instructed by the physician. Do not take more than the dose prescribed. Chronic abuse of stimulants can lead to tolerance and dependence and, potentially, addictive behavior.
- Do not crush or chew the long-acting stimulants. Do not open the capsules unless instructed to do so.
- It is recommended that methylphenidate be taken about one-half hour before meals.
- Take the last daily dose early in the evening around 6 P.M. to avoid insomnia.

Use of Alcohol and Other Medications

Patients should not consume alcohol, since it may exacerbate the symptoms of ADHD. Some medications, including over-the-counter medicines, may interact with stimulants, and they should not be taken concomitantly. The drug interaction may *lower* the blood level of the affected drug and decrease the drug's effectiveness; or, it may *elevate* the blood level of the affected drug and cause toxicity. For example, methylphenidate may increase the blood levels of anticonvulsants, such as phenytoin (Dilantin), resulting in possible toxic effects. Diet pills should not be taken with stimulants because the combination may result in excessive central nervous system stimulation, leading to agitation, anxiety, and psychosis. Be cautious of using other medications with stimulant properties. These include decongestants, which may be found in cold and allergy medications sold over-the-counter, and certain inhalers used for breathing, such as albuterol (Ventolin). Stimulants should *never* be taken with antidepressants known as **monoamine oxidase inhibitors** (MAOIs). Taking these two medications together may result in dangerous elevation of blood pressure.

POSSIBLE SIDE EFFECTS

Adjusting the dose or switching to an extended-release stimulant may manage the following frequent side effects of stimulants:

- Reduced appetite
- Weight loss
- Delay of sleep onset and insomnia
- Jitteriness and nervousness
- Headaches
- Palpitations and rapid heart rate
- Rebound effect (the child may become mildly irritable or hyperactive when the stimulant wears off)

POSSIBLE ADVERSE REACTIONS

- *Drug dependence.* Stimulants, particularly the amphetamines, have a high potential for abuse. Individuals with a history of alcohol and substance abuse may be at risk for abusing stimulants. Stimulant abusers increase the amount they take many times over the treatment dosages. Signs of abuse include marked insomnia, increased energy and hyperactivity, personality changes, poor concentration, disorganized thoughts, and compulsive behavior. With extended intoxication and sleepless nights, the individual may manifest psychotic symptoms. Abusers develop tolerance of and psychological dependence to stimulants that result in the social disabilities of addiction.

- *Growth suppression.* Stimulants are associated with suppression of linear growth in children and adolescents. Physicians commonly interrupt the medication on weekends and holidays when children are not in school for growth catch-up. Use of stimulants during the adolescent years must be carefully considered by the physician with the patient and family to determine the benefits and risk of treatment.

- *Tics (twitching).* In patients with tic disorder (i.e., twitching of a muscle group, especially in the face), stimulants may make tics worse. Some children with no previous history may develop tics during treatment with stimulants. When stimulants are stopped, tic movements subside.

- *Elevation of blood pressure.* Stimulants may increase blood pressure. Generally, blood pressure is increased mild to moderately by stimulants. Patients should be checked routinely while taking stimulants. Patients with severe high blood pressure should not take stimulants.

PREGNANCY AND BREAST FEEDING

The amphetamines and methylphenidate are in **Category C** of the U.S. Food and Drug Administration (FDA) Pregnancy Risk Categories. Placement in this category indicates that stimulants have been found to produce birth defects in animals, but there are insufficient data to determine the risk in humans. However, the risks of using stimulants during pregnancy may be inferred from infants born to mothers dependent on amphetamines, who are premature and of low birth weight. These infants also show signs of withdrawal after birth.

Amphetamines are excreted in breast milk, but it is not known whether methylphenidate is found in human milk. It is recommended that mothers not use stimulants if they desire to breastfeed.

If you have any questions about this handout, please consult your physician.

INFORMATION ABOUT

COGNITIVE ENHANCERS

FOR PATIENTS AND FAMILIES

○ **Donepezil (Aricept)**   ○ **Rivastigmine (Exelon)**

○ **Galantamine (Reminyl)**   ○ **Tacrine (Cognex)**

○ **Memantine (Namenda)**

Cognitive enhancers are medications used for treatment of mild to moderate dementia of Alzheimer's type. Alzheimer's disease is a progressive and irreversible deterioration of the brain with loss of mental capacity, and it is the most common cause of dementia in the elderly. The cause of Alzheimer's disease is unknown, but manifestations of the disease are due in part to the selective loss of brain cells known as **cholinergic neurons** in certain areas of the brain. It is believed that memory loss in Alzheimer's patients is due to deterioration of these cholinergic neurons. Agents known as cognitive enhancers promote the function of these neurons by inhibiting the breakdown of their neurotransmitter, **acetylcholine.** By inhibiting acetylcholine destruction (by blocking the **cholinesterase** enzyme that breaks down acetylcholine), these agents enhance the function of cholinergic neurons. Alzheimer's patients may benefit from cognitive enhancers and exhibit improvement in their memory and other areas of cognitive function, especially during the early stages of the disease.

Memantine (Namenda) was recently approved to treat moderate to severe Alzheimer's disease. Unlike the other cognitive enhancers, memantine works by a different mechanism of action. Instead of blocking cholinesterase and increasing acetylcholine, memantine antagonizes the action of **glutamate**, an excitatory neurotransmitter, which plays an important role in learning and memory. Researchers believe that in Alzheimer's disease, the activity of glutamate is not regulated correctly, and this then leads to overexcitation and death of nerve cells. Evidence shows that memantine works by attaching to a specific site on glutamate receptors in the brain, thus modulating the activity of glutamate so that the right amount is available.

The benefits of these agents in improving cognitive function in Alzheimer's disease may be highly variable among patients. The best responders are usually patients in the early stages when the disease has not taken its toll and a relatively larger number of cholinergic neurons are still intact compared with during the later stages. As the patient's disease advances, further destruction of cholinergic neurons removes target sites for acetylcholine to exert its action, and these agents then offer little benefit. The usual response, however, does not always predict an individual response. It may require a trial with several agents to determine if the patient will benefit from a cognitive enhancer. Studies have shown that patients who do not respond to one cognitive enhancer may respond adequately to another.

When patients respond to cognitive enhancers, they may show robust improvement in memory and overall cognitive ability. Unfortunately, these agents do not arrest the ravages of the disease. With time, patients will be at the stage where they were before beginning the drug and then continue on a downhill decline when these agents may no longer be effective.

HOW THESE MEDICATIONS ARE PRESCRIBED

Tacrine (Cognex) was the first cognitive enhancer released in the United States for enhancement of memory in Alzheimer's disease. The drug is associated with liver toxicity, and liver function tests must be monitored routinely while taking the medication. The usual dose for the first 4 weeks is 10 mg four times daily (40 mg/day), administered at least 1 hour before meals. After 4 weeks of treatment at this dosage, and if there is no sign of liver problems, the dose may be increased to 20 mg four times a day (80 mg/day). The dosage may be further increased by 40 mg/day at 4- to 6-week intervals if the drug is tolerated and there is no liver toxicity, to a maximum dosage of 160 mg/day.

Donepezil (Aricept) requires only once-a-day dosing, just prior to bedtime. The starting dose is 5 mg at bedtime. Most patients can be maintained at this dosage, but some patients may do better with a daily dose of 10 mg. However, patients should not have their drug increased to 10 mg until they have been at 5 mg for 5–6 weeks.

Rivastigmine (Exelon) is dosed twice a day, in the morning and evening, and should be taken with food. The starting dose is 1.5 mg twice a day (3 mg/day). Depending on the patient's tolerance, the dose may be increased after 2 weeks to 3 mg twice a day (6 mg/day). The dose may be increased further by 3 mg daily every 2 weeks to a maximum dose of 6 mg twice daily (12 mg/day).

Galantamine (Reminyl) is also administered twice a day, preferably in the morning and evening with meals. The usual starting dose is 4 mg twice daily (8 mg/day). The dose may be increased after 4 weeks to 8 mg twice daily (16 mg/day), depending on the patient's tolerability. If needed, further increases are made after 4-week intervals. The recommended dosage range is 16 to 24 mg/day, with the medication administered twice daily.

The starting dose for **memantine** (Namenda) is 5 mg a day for the first week; in week 2, the dose is increased to 5 mg two times a day; in week 3, the dose is increased to 15 mg/day (10 mg in the morning and 5 mg at bedtime); and by week 4, the target dosage of 20 mg/day is attained (10 mg two times a day thereafter). This titration schedule, of course, depends on the patient's tolerability to the dose of the medication.

PROPER USE OF THESE MEDICATIONS:
INSTRUCTIONS FOR PATIENTS AND CAREGIVERS

Storing Your Medication

- Keep the medication in a tamper-resistant vial and out of reach of children (or the patient). Overdosage with these medications is very hazardous.
- Store the medication so as to keep it from excessive heat, moisture, and direct light.
- Keep the medication in its original prescription vial with the label intact to prevent someone from taking medication inadvertently.

Taking Your Medication

- Take the medication exactly as instructed by the physician. Do not take more than the dose prescribed. Take or administer the medication at regular intervals. This is especially important with tacrine, which must be taken four times daily. Tacrine should be taken at least 1 hour before meals. The other agents may be taken with food to avoid an upset stomach.
- If you miss a dose, take it as soon as possible. However, if it is near the time of the next dose, skip the dose you missed and go back to the regular dosing schedule, but do not double-up the dose.
- Do not abruptly discontinue the medication or reduce the dose without consulting with the physician. This may cause a decline in cognitive function and behavior changes. The medication should never be increased unless instructed by your physician.

Use of Alcohol and Other Medications

Patients taking cognitive enhancer medications should not use alcohol. Alcohol, which is a depressant, not only negates the benefits of the medication, but may further compromise cognitive function.

Some medications, including over-the-counter medicines, may interact with cognitive enhancers and therefore should not be taken concomitantly. The drug interaction may *lower* the blood level of the affected drug and decrease the drug's effectiveness; or, it may *elevate* the blood level of the affected drug and cause toxicity. Inform the physician of all prescription and over-the-counter medications the patient is taking. If the patient or caretaker has questions about the medications, consult a physician or pharmacist.

POSSIBLE SIDE EFFECTS

- *Gastrointestinal (GI) side effects.* GI side effects include nausea, vomiting, diarrhea, heartburn, and loss of appetite. These side effects are the most frequent complaints and reasons for discontinuation of these agents. Cognitive enhancers may increase gastric acid secretion, so that patients with a history of ulcers should be aware of signs of gastrointestinal bleeding.
- *Weight loss with rivastigmine.* Patients taking rivastigmine at high dosages (9 mg/day or higher) may experience significant weight loss, which may or may not be associated with loss of appetite, nausea, vomiting, or diarrhea. Women taking rivastigmine are more prone to weight loss than are men.
- *Dizziness, headaches, confusion, and incoordination.* If there is a rapid and sudden change in patient's mental status or behavior, the family member or caregiver should contact the physician.
- *Exacerbation of pulmonary* diseases. Patients with a history of asthma or chronic lung disease should be aware that these agents might make their symptoms worse.

POSSIBLE ADVERSE REACTIONS

- *Liver toxicity.* Approximately 50% of patients treated with tacrine (Cognex) developed a slight elevation of liver enzyme levels. A smaller percentage of these patients will have markedly elevated liver enzymes, which is indicative of liver cell damage. Patients with mild to moderately elevated liver enzymes usually do not have any symptoms. When liver function is markedly compromised, the patient may manifest symptoms that include flulike symptoms, tiredness, loss of appetite, and jaundice (yellow coloration of the skin and whites of the eyes because the liver cannot process one of its byproducts, bilirubin). Because of tacrine's potential for liver toxicity, physicians obtain blood tests to monitor liver enzyme levels every other week for the first 16 weeks, and then every 3 months thereafter. If the patient's enzyme level is two times the upper limit of normal, the dose for tacrine is reduced, and if it is five times the upper limit of normal, the medication is discontinued.
- *Lower heart rate and blood pressure.* These agents may lower heart rate and blood pressure. Elderly patient and patients with a history of cardiac conduction problems should be particularly cautious of the potential of this adverse reaction. Fainting episodes have also been reported with use of these agents.
- *Increased memantine blood levels with alkaline urine and renal impairment.* Because memantine is eliminated primarily by the kidneys, severe renal impairment may diminish excretion of the drug and elevate blood levels, resulting in possible toxicity. Furthermore, conditions that make the urine more alkaline (i.e., raise urine pH) may decrease excretion of memantine and raise blood levels. The urine may be made more alkaline by diet, drugs (c.g., sodium bicarbonate), and medical conditions (e.g., severe urinary tract infection).

If you have any questions about this handout, please consult your physician.

References

American Psychiatric Association: Diagnostic and Statistical Manual of Mental Disorders, 4th Edition, Text Revision. Washington, DC, American Psychiatric Association, 2000

Andreasen NC, Black DW: Introductory Textbook of Psychiatry, 3rd Edition. Washington, DC, American Psychiatric Publishing, 2001

Hales RE, Hales D: The Mind/Mood Pill Book. New York, Bantam Books, 2000

Hales RE, Yudofsky SC (eds): The American Psychiatric Publishing Textbook of Clinical Psychiatry, 4th Edition. Washingon, DC, American Psychiatric Publishing, 2003

Janicak PG, Davis JM, Preskorn SH, et al: Principles and Practice of Psychopharmacotherapy, 3rd Edition. Philadelphia, PA, Lippincott Williams & Wilkins, 2001

Kaplan HI, Sadock BJ, Grebb JA: Kaplan and Sadock's Synopsis of Psychiatry: Behavioral Sciences/Clinical Psychiatry, 9th Edition. Philadelphia, PA, Lippincott Williams & Wilkins, 2002

Index